Building Healthy Communities

Related Titles

Principles and Foundations of Health Promotion and Education
Randall R. Cottrell, James T. Girvan, and James F. McKenzie
ISBN: 0-205-27365-3

Planning, Implementing, and Evaluating Health Promotion Programs: A Primer, Second Edition
James F. McKenzie and Jan L. Smeltzer
ISBN: 0-205-20069-9

Community Health in the 21st Century
Patricia A. Reagan and Jodi Brookins-Fisher
ISBN: 0-205-19749-3

Building Healthy Communities

The Challenge of Health Care in the Twenty-First Century

Edited by

Annette J. McBeth

Immanuel St. Joseph's–Mayo Health System
Mankato, Minnesota

Kathryn D. Schweer

Allen College, Waterloo, Iowa

Allyn and Bacon

Boston ▪ London ▪ Toronto ▪ Sydney ▪ Tokyo ▪ Singapore

Publisher: *Joseph E. Burns*
Series Editorial Assistant: *Sue Walther Jones*
Manufacturing Buyer: *David Repetto*
Marketing Manager: *Richard Muhr*

A Pearson Education Company
Needham Heights, MA 02494

Internet: www.abacon.com

Library of Congress Cataloging-in-Publication Data

Building healthy communities : the challenge of health care in the twenty-first century / Annette J. McBeth, Kathryn D. Schweer, editors.
p. cm.
Includes bibliographical references and index.
ISBN 0-205-27618-0
1. Health planning—United States. 2. Medical care—United States—Forecasting. 3. Medical policy—United States—Forecasting. I. McBeth, Annette J. II. Schweer, Kathryn D.
RA395.A3B845 1999
362.1'0973'0905—dc21 99-35784
CIP

Printed in the United States of America
10 9 8 7 6 5 4 3 2 1 04 03 02 01 00

To those who are building healthy communities today for the children of tomorrow.

CONTENTS

FOREWORD

Imagine an integrated, holistic health system that serves people throughout their lifespan. Imagine achieving not just the vision but the reality of healthy people living in healthy communities. This book gives the reader a template of how we can achieve healthy people by *"Building Healthy Communities."*

Jonas Salk, MD, said "We are no longer our own niche. We must see ourselves as part of the ecosystem." Martin Luther King, Jr., said, "We are caught in an inescapable network of mutuality, tied into a single garment of destiny."

The implications and significance of these two quotes could have been the basic inspiration for McBeth and Schweer. These two primary authors clearly understand what Salk and King are saying—that all humans are connected to each other, to their communities, and to their environment. These authors have done a splendid job of combining the efforts of eleven other health care professionals who elucidate in just nine chapters how a better balance can be achieved between our present, powerful, disease care system and the community primary health care model that is so needed for the future.

The authors do not at all suggest that there is any reason to abandon the present system of disease care. It fulfills a most important need. But they also seem to fully agree with the words of Ronald David, MD, Chief Medical Officer of D.C. Health and Hospitals Public Benefit Corporation in Washington, D.C. "We tend to seek medical solutions to what are essentially tears in the social fabric. These tears can be in terms of violence, economic oppression and class ostracism, racism, sexism, and a whole host of factors." Dr. David goes on to say, "Health is a capacity to adapt and evolve toward ever more complex and creative wholes. It is a capacity that can only be realized in the context of mutually supportive human relationships."

Dr. David will surely love reading this book because what *Building Healthy Communities* is about is explaining how people in each community can deal with "tears in the social fabric" through "mutually supportive human relationships" done through the context of the community primary health care model.

What happens in most communities when a disaster such as a flood, a tornado, or a meningitis outbreak occurs? Usually, there is an incredible outpouring of collaboration and mutually supportive human relationships. Organizations, institutions, and businesses that have been competitive become collaborative. These groups begin to work together sharing their vision in a planning process that is uniquely noncompetitive. There is usually a sharing of accountability plus a partnering of these disparate groups. There is a movement away from the needs and demands of individuals to what can best be described as the needs of the entire community. This is what the community primary health care model is about, and **it is the core of what this book is about.** This model and this book say that by paying attention to not only health services but also to economics, politics, environment, agriculture/nutrition, and education, the health of the community and, therefore, individuals will be improved.

Few people would argue that we Americans do a good job of collaborating and providing relief from acute disasters such as floods and tornadoes. Most would also agree that we have a long way to go to improve our handling of the chronic disasters that Dr. David calls the "tears in the social fabric." The increasing amount of violence, abuse issues, economic oppression, racism, and forty-five million Americans with no medical insurance coverage are affecting the quality of life for every citizen of this country. How do the authors suggest mobilizing the collaborative energy and citizen enthusiasm that is so evident at the time of acute disasters to be responsive on a long-term basis to these more chronic disasters or tears in the social fabric?

This book presents a very readable guide of how the community primary health care model can be developed. Like many brilliant plans, this one is quite simple in design. It does require the difficult task of changing established patterns of competition, control, and power. The book describes how to change these patterns by explaining how this new community health care model can best be used. The model imitates the things that work so well in acute disasters and uses those same ideas to help solve the ongoing tears in our social fabric—the chronic disasters. Two examples will illustrate this point.

- The new community primary health care model works collaboratively on an ongoing basis to promote health and healing for *all* citizens so as to eliminate the chronic disaster of 45 million uninsured Americans. That plan imitates how we now respond to an acute disaster such as a flood or tornado in which *every* affected citizen gets assistance, not just those who can afford it.
- The new model links private, government, and community-based organizations in an interactive planning process to create a shared vision of how to help eliminate some of the chronic disasters such as violence that we have come to accept as normal. The model again imitates how after an acute disaster (a tornado) representative groups come together and decide what steps will work best to solve the problem. In other words, they do interactive planning with the sharing of visions regarding how to best accomplish the required tasks necessary to solve the problem.

Many Americans believe it is now a time in our history that presents us with the paradox of being both the best of times and the worst of times. There is among many a feeling that much of the violence, sickness, and death in America is linked to a loneliness, to a breakdown of human bonds, and to not feeling a sense of community. This book, *Building Healthy Communities,* is the best antidote I know of to reverse the factors causing the worst of our times. After reading it, it is not hard to imagine an integrated, holistic health system serving healthy people who are living in healthy communities—truly living in the best of times.

Bill Manahan, M.D.
Assistant Professor
Department of Family Practice and Community Health
Academic Health Center
University of Minnesota
Minneapolis, Minnesota

PREFACE

Health care in the twenty-first century must move beyond a focus on access, quality, and cost of care to a broader vision of building healthy communities. Leaders in health care service and education, together with other organizational, community, and governmental leaders, will benefit from sharing perspectives and creating strategies for improving people's health and building healthy communities. When a community has discovered its shared values, and when its members are committed to working together in partnerships, that community will be able to use its expertise to shape a healthy future.

Building Healthy Communities: The Challenge of Health Care in the Twenty-First Century is not intended to be a textbook or a review of literature on health care delivery. Instead, it focuses on achieving the vision of healthy people and healthy communities. The information presented herein emerged as people embraced certain models and frameworks. One pervading framework is that if everyone participates in a learning organization, new and better ways of working together are launched.

In Chapter 1, the importance of working to integrate health care services is discussed. Efforts to meet community health needs are most successful in an atmosphere of trust and respect. Health care providers must work collaboratively with the community to achieve the health, healing, and wholeness that Florence Nightingale espoused in the nineteenth century.

As outlined in Chapter 2, the process of building healthy communities evolved from *The Surgeon General's Report of Health Promotion and Disease Prevention* (1979) to a proposed framework as cited in *Healthy People 2010* (1997). The interactive planning process is useful for creating change in complex social systems. It is based on two essential concepts: systems thinking and design. Education and training in use of the interactive planning process will enable a community to design and build its own vision for a healthy community.

Chapter 3 focuses on ways in which people and agencies from a nine-county area learned to work together to accommodate social, political, economic, and technical forces challenging health care. A population-based and community-based approach requires involvement of all stakeholders, especially the consumer. Identification and achievement of regional health goals will result.

The importance of a shared vision is the theme of Chapter 4. Several examples of the processes used to achieve a shared vision are described, and outcomes are presented.

The health care delivery system of the twenty-first century demands a culture change at all levels. In Chapter 5, a community primary health care model built upon community need and choice improves health outcomes. Examples are presented to demonstrate the effect of culture change.

In Chapter 6, the imperative of a continuum of care is described. Alternatives to fragmented, duplicated, and wasteful use of health care services are illustrated in three case scenarios. Providing health services that meet the needs of people throughout the life span, at all stages of the health–illness continuum, and in all settings requires creative and innovative strategies for providing a continuum of care.

Chapter 7 describes quality evaluation as a young science. The need for quality measurement in health care has never been greater. The challenge for the twenty-first century will be to develop and apply measures that can distinguish true quality differences. Success will depend on cooperative efforts to advance this young science.

Chapter 8 emphasizes the importance of creating an ongoing learning organization able to shape its own future. An important outcome of service–education partnerships is the creation of quality, cost-effective, accessible education for practice in the work world. The goal of building healthy communities for people in the twenty-first century can best be accomplished through partnerships.

The challenges ahead of us in the twenty-first century are outlined in Chapter 9. Meshing the values of the people in our communities with the values of health care providers is essential if the challenges are to be met successfully. Setting goals focused on the health of people and communities is a unifying force. Managing change, networking with community builders, preparing leaders for new roles, and using the latest innovations in information technology are strategies for achieving these goals. Three of the many possible directions for health care are (1) implementation of holistic preventive guidelines, (2) complementary and/or alternative therapies, and (3) collegial collaboration for primary care services. Each community is encouraged to explore its own ways to attain healthy people and healthy communities.

When we first met, we were relatively new to our positions as vice president of a medium-sized regional community hospital and dean of a school of nursing at a comprehensive state university. Affiliations between the hospital and nursing school had existed for over forty years. There were many positive connections between the two institutions. However, as newcomers, we were unfamiliar with both history and the potential for meeting the challenge of health care. We had been meeting informally over dinner, once a month, when a request for proposals from The Robert Wood Johnson Foundation/Pew Charitable Trust initiative, "Strengthening Hospital Nursing: A Program to Improve Patient Care," came to the vice president of the hospital, and our journey of discovery began. As we moved forward, leaders from two rural community hospitals and the local technical college joined us. This leadership group became energized by a shared vision of meeting the health needs of individuals and families through a regionally integrated health and education system.

In describing our journey, we have highlighted the risks we took, discoveries we made, what worked and what did not work, and what guiding principles evolved. We ask you to consider the unique challenges of health care during the transition into the twenty-first century. We trust that what we have learned from our journey will give you insights about building bridges and systems within your organization, community, and region in order to make your communities healthy places in which to work and live in the twenty-first century.

Annette J. McBeth
Kathryn D. Schweer

References

U.S. Department of Health and Human Services (1997). Developing objectives for healthy people 2010. Washington, D.C.: Health and Human Services, Office of Disease Prevention and Health Promotion.

U.S. Institute of Medicine (1979). *Healthy People: The Surgeon General's report on health promotion and disease prevention.* Washington, D.C., U.S. Government Printing Office.

ACKNOWLEDGMENTS

Facilitator and Coordinator of Book Manuscript Preparation

John A. Romas, M.P.H., Ph.D.
Professor, Department of Health Science
Minnesota State University, Mankato,*
Mankato, MN

Administrative Assistant
Catherine Maczuga
Immanuel St. Joseph's-Mayo Health System
Mankato, Minnesota

Technical Writing Consultants

Robert Mehltretter
North Mankato, MN

Kristin Woizeschke, M.L.S.
Health Resource Librarian
Immanuel St. Joseph's–Mayo Health System
Mankato, MN

Leadership Writing Team

Annette J. McBeth, R.N., M.S., F.A.A.N.
Vice President
Immanuel St. Joseph's–Mayo Health System
Mankato, MN

Kathryn D. Schweer, R.N., Ph.D.
Professor and Dean of Academic Affairs
Allen College
Waterloo, IA

Sharon P. Aadelen, Ph.D., R.N.
Professor, School of Nursing
Minnesota State University, Mankato
Mankato, MN

Jerome A. Crest, M.H.A.
Executive Vice President
Immanuel St. Joseph's–Mayo Health System
Mankato, MN

Laurie Dahl, R.N., M.P.H.
Director, Community Health Services
Immanuel St. Joseph's–Mayo Health System
Mankato, MN

Lynette Froehlich, R.N.
Senior Nurse Manager
Hutchinson Hospital
Burns Manor Nursing Home
Hutchinson, MN

Mary Kay Hohenstein, R.N., M.Ed.
Former Health Coordinator, South Central Technical College
North Mankato, MN
Former Director of Nursing Continuing Education
Minnesota State University, Mankato
Mankato, MN

*Name change effective 1998; formerly Mankato State University.

Kay Hubbard
Director of Quality Resources
Immanuel St. Joseph's–Mayo Health System
Mankato, MN

Mary I. Huntley, R.N., Ph.D.
Professor, School of Nursing
Minnesota State University, Mankato
Mankato, MN

Kristin Juliar, M.A.
Project Coordinator
Healthcare Education–Industry Partnership
Minnesota State University, Mankato
Mankato, MN

Shirley Raetz, R.N.
Director of Patient Support Services
Waseca Medical Center
Waseca, MN

Alice Weydt, R.N., M.S.
Director, Patient Care Services
Immanuel St. Joseph's–Mayo Health System
Mankato, MN

Douglas L. Wood, M.D.
Vice Chair, Department of Internal Medicine
Mayo Clinic
Rochester, MN

Book Reviewers

Laurie Dahl, R.N., M.P.H.
Director, Community Health Services
Immanuel St. Joseph's–Mayo Health System
Mankato, MN

Mary I. Huntley, R.N., Ph.D.
Professor, School of Nursing
Minnesota State University, Mankato
Mankato, MN

Kristin Juliar, M.A.
Project Coordinator
Healthcare Education–Industry Partnership
Minnesota State University, Mankato
Mankato, MN

Bill Manahan, M.D.
Assistant Professor, Department of Family Practice and Community Health
Academic Health Center
University of Minnesota
Minneapolis, MN

James F. McKenzie, Ph.D., M.P.H.
Professor, Department of Physiology and Health Science
Ball State University
Muncie, IN

Thomas W. O'Rourke, M.P.H., Ph.D.
Professor, Community Health
University of Illinois
Champaign–Urbana, IL

John A. Romas, M.P.H., Ph.D.
Professor, Department of Health Science
Minnesota State University
Mankato, MN

Alice Weydt, R.N., M.S.
Director, Patient Care Services
Immanuel St. Joseph's–Mayo Health System
Mankato, MN

Douglas L. Wood, M.D.
Vice Chair, Department of Internal Medicine
Mayo Clinic
Rochester, MN

FIGURES AND TABLES

Building Healthy Communities

CHAPTER

1 Moving Forward to the Twenty-First Century

DOUGLAS L. WOOD
ANNETTE J. McBETH
KATHRYN D. SCHWEER

> Florence Nightingale's vision more than a century ago... *to minister to whole beings with tender loving care and to create an environment in which the patient [client] can find healing...*
>
> —Florence Nightingale, 1860

- Current Problems in Health Care
- Integrated Delivery Systems
- Managed Care and Community Health
- A Strategy for Government Programs
- Education for the Future
- Summary

Rapid changes in the organization of health care delivery in the United States during the last decade of the twentieth century have created public uneasiness about the future of health care. Many community-based nonprofit hospitals have been converted to for-profit entities and merged with large delivery systems. It is natural to be concerned about whether the best interests of people needing health care may be compromised by the increasing commercialization of health care.

Some argue that these concerns are a result of actions by managed care organizations, large hospitals, or physician management organizations. However, problems with fee-for-service medicine also contribute to declining public trust in health care. Overutilization of tests and procedures in fee-for-service settings is as much a matter of concern as is underutilization in certain managed care settings.

Amid the controversy surrounding these changes, there is concern about community health care and the need to help protect the underserved population while reducing overall health care costs. Effective community care is more likely to be accomplished by integration of multiple delivery systems than by managed care. Government control of managed care would not assure that the uninsured and underinsured in our communities receive adequate health care.

Physicians, hospitals, and health plans will need to work in a cooperative and coordinated manner with consumers and providers in order to assure both individual and community health. Because resources available for this task (both public and private dollars) are limited, it is necessary to form collaborative partnerships. At the local, state, and national level, our society must be willing to shift more of its health care dollars to population-based approaches focused on promoting health. Examples are like those advocated in *Healthy People 2010* (U.S. Department of Health and Human Services, 1997).

Current Problems in Health Care

Health care in the United States is expensive. Though increases in health care spending have slowed recently, medical care costs are still increasing. Utilization of resources continues to rise exponentially. Use of expensive new drugs and technology without careful evaluation of effectiveness contributes to overall expense. Despite increasing medical care outlays, performance and quality outcomes remain uneven across the country and within communities. Physicians, providers, and payers seek to minimize risk through careful selection of patients.

Performance variations occur even in markets that are considered to be mature managed care environments. The development of disease management strategies illustrates the significant duplication of resources that occurs during hospitalization or during the movement of the patient from one provider system to another. Our present health care delivery system is not functioning as a system. Consequently, users are confronted by frustrating fragmentation and costly inefficiencies.

In hospitals, competition and business pressure are reducing profit margins. Cost shifting to private payers to subsidize losses has reached its limits. Continued reductions in federal and state (i.e., Medicare and Medicaid) payments to hospitals and providers will cause hospital cost growth to outpace revenue growth and will mean that hospitals will have less money for charity care and other community-based activities. Corporations and private purchasers are reluctant to continue to support cost shifting since they have been successful in reducing the rate of growth in their own health spending.

Society seeks to derive maximum benefit from those resources committed to health care and to minimize the economic and social costs associated with the provision of health care services. Increased limitation on availability of resources from government and private sources creates a series of conflicts for decision makers. The needs of society must be weighed against the needs (or wants) of individuals and/or businesses. Increasingly difficult decisions between cost and quality will have to be made.

Decision makers, hospitals, health care providers, and the public must confront basic value conflicts in addressing the direction of future health care delivery. These conflicts include

- The commitment to high-quality care while controlling costs
- Investment in public health programs that promote individual responsibility rather than directing more resources to care of the sick
- Diverting more funds to health promotion and prevention activities while providing illness care to all who need it
- Addressing societal wishes for quality, cost-effective, accessible health care
- Providing needed care in each community while dealing with unrealistic "wants," such as utilization of the latest technology.

It will be necessary to find strategies to resolve these value conflicts in a cost-effective manner. Individuals and families will need to be motivated to use the health promotion and disease prevention services made available to them by their communities. Providers must help consumers learn to practice healthful behaviors. Elimination of current problems in health care will also require effective integration of delivery systems. Information systems and communication networks must be developed to facilitate movement of patients from one provider to another or one system to another without the inefficiencies and fragmentation that characterize current systems.

Integrated Delivery Systems

In most communities, multiple health care providers, hospitals, self-insured companies, and a variety of payers will have to learn to work as partners to care for the community. Working together can best be done in an integrated manner. An integrated delivery system is a patient-oriented system of care that spans all levels of care. It is comprised of services and integrated mechanisms that guide and track patients over time through a comprehensive array of holistic health and social services. In an integrated delivery system, formal arrangements and common financial incentives exist among all providers, payers, and consumers of health care. This does not require a single financing mechanism or a single governance system. It does require cooperation, coordination, common goals, and strong leadership that is committed to a systems approach.

The primary goal of an integrated health care delivery system is healthy people in a healthy community. Other goals include high-quality care, appropriate utilization of tests and treatments, economic efficiency, and consumer, staff, and payer satisfaction. The development of systems that can achieve these goals requires a merger of some provider organizations, integration of physician practices, development of practice and referral guidelines, and an emphasis on the needs of the consumer with a strong commitment to assuring continuity of care between providers and systems. This integration can result in a reduction in acute-care beds, a redeployment of clinical services, including case management services, and design of a new regionally integrated delivery system focusing on health.

The successful integrated delivery system of the twenty-first century will be characterized by superior service, high quality, and competitive pricing. Comprehensive services will be available across a continuum of care. Information systems will provide the mechanism to communicate and evaluate care in a clinically relevant and meaningful manner. Providers and other components of the system will be able to use the information to improve care processes. The integrated delivery system will successfully achieve financial goals, including generating capital for system growth and development. Finally, trust and cohesiveness among providers, consumers, purchasers, and payers will sustain community confidence in the delivery system.

There are significant challenges to successful implementation of such an integrated delivery system. Before an integrated delivery system can be successful, there must be effective leadership that is committed to what Senge (1990) refers to as systems thinking orientation. Courageous leadership may be needed to arrive at decisions that do not favor a particular leader, institution, or group. The incentive for success will have to be oriented to the system rather than to individuals or institutions.

Current efforts to integrate health care delivery have included mergers and partnerships such as preferred-provider organizations (PPOs) and health maintenance organizations (HMOs). These organizations have established ways to provide managed care. Collaborative efforts among all HMOs and other health care providers will be needed to build healthier communities.

Managed Care and Community Health

The population-based orientation of managed care includes community-based or employment-based enrollment and a financing mechanism that allows more innovation than does fee-for-service medicine. This orientation has created an expectation that managed care organizations will be more successful in achieving improvements in community health than in other aspects of health care. Most managed care organizations are oriented to the population composed of their members rather than the population of the community as a whole. However, there are examples of significant community orientation among nonprofit HMOs in some parts of the country.

Although concerns exist about some parts of managed care, especially in how clinical decisions may be influenced by physician compensation arrangements, managed care organizations are more oriented to providing information about provider performance and patient outcomes than are other delivery systems. Such organizations are more likely to participate in efforts that improve public health than are traditional organizations. Finally, a commitment to data-driven improvement of practice to achieve superior outcomes is more common among managed care organizations. Such organizations are faster to adopt disease management strategies and other efforts to better utilize precious resources. Thus, managed care organizations are in a strategic position to improve the health status of a community. However, success in this endeavor also depends on a systems orientation, a willingness to respond to the public's expressed needs, and the ability to work collaboratively with other managed care organizations as well as other health care providers within the community.

So far, managed care organizations have failed to make significant contributions to community health because they have been focused on serving populations determined by employer mix or competition in the marketplace. The likelihood that federal and state governments may seek more managed care options for care of persons on Medicare or Medicaid, chronically disabled populations, and large blocks of government employees creates a new opportunity for managed care organizations to focus on building healthy communities. Working in an integrated manner with government health and human service agencies to provide a combination of health care and other services can result in improved community health status.

There are four potential barriers to achieving success in improving community health when Medicare and Medicaid are converted to managed care. First, governments have little or no experience in managing risk and providing allocation of resources to health care. Second, there may be little or no additional money to provide community services, since governments are seeking ways to reduce overall health care spending. Third, there is a possibility that local government units may see federal block grants and state payment reforms as a new revenue source for social programs, effectively reducing the number of dollars available for community health initiatives. Fourth, because federal bailouts are not available under the terms of new programs, providers are at risk of not being paid if government funds are exhausted before the end of the term of a contract.

The number of populations needing care will produce intense pressure on funding sources for government programs. A commitment of dollars will be required for numerous programs, including basic health care coverage for the uninsured and underinsured, care for the chronically disabled, detoxification and chemical dependency services, long-term nursing care, and care for immigrant or other special interest groups.

Thus, in a setting of significant budget constraints, Medicare and Medicaid managed care will necessitate keeping administrative costs at the lowest possible level, recruiting providers, and sharing risk with other populations, especially government employees. Integrated delivery systems are in a strong position to implement strategies to effectively serve the needs of government, which include providing health care services for underinsured and uninsured community members.

A Strategy for Government Programs

As integrated health systems are formed, strategies for managed care have been developed that include governmental health care programs. An example of how one system approaches this opportunity is described below.

The Mayo Health System has evaluated its potential for providing services to governmental programs. In its approach to managed care, the Mayo Health System strives to understand the needs and concerns of local governments and develop products that can be delivered in an integrated delivery system. The goal is to satisfy the needs of government payers and consumers while reducing the risk to providers.

Effective communication with local officials and community business leaders is an important part of success for such programs. Mayo Health System principles for managed care include, but are not limited to, the following elements:

- Promote dedication to patient care and quality
- Respect the physician-patient relationship
- Provide leadership support for physicians and other team leaders
- Keep medical management at a minimum; use an interdisciplinary team approach
- Contract as a system, and avoid separating specific populations, such as behavioral health or chronic renal disease, from the managed care plan
- Facilitate consistency in medical management, reporting, and information systems
- Work in partnership with local government units
- Develop products in anticipation of market needs
- Utilize information systems to support achievement of superior results
- Maximize dollars available for patient care through efficient administration
- Pay providers equitably
- Require consistency in payment terms among payers and sites

Education for the Future

In order to achieve an integrated health care delivery system, health care providers need to prepare themselves for collaborative, interdisciplinary approaches. For some physicians, nurses, and other allied health professionals, a paradigm shift may be required. The old paradigm of the physician in control of an individual's care must give way to a community perspective that uses the full potential of the knowledge and skills of all providers. In order to meet the goal of quality, cost-effective care, interdisciplinary teams must work together to determine the level of care required for an individual, family, or community group, and then decide who is best qualified to deliver care in each situation. Lasker (1997) reported the discovery of more than five hundred examples of collaborations from a series of focus groups with students and practitioners from different disciplines throughout the country. In most cases, the health care professionals did not know where to begin because they had so little experience in collaboration. However, when events such as disease epidemics, the emergence of managed care, and consolidation of public and private services begin to affect health care in a community, providers have strong incentives to learn new ways of working together.

Lasker (1997) has also noted that when medical and public health professionals with resources available in institutions combine their skills, synergies are developed. Some of the synergies discovered in collaboration include (1) providing a framework for health care for the uninsured; (2) coordinating health care services available to individuals; (3) applying epidemiological models to improve the quality and cost-effectiveness of care; (4) adapting clinical practice successes to achieve public health goals; (5) bringing diverse community groups together to deal with such health issues as smoking, substance abuse, violence, and domestic abuse; and (6) shaping the work environment to include both the individual and community health perspectives.

Health care professionals currently in practice have difficulty learning how to function in an integrated health care delivery system. Students have the even more formidable task of learning both their own discipline and other disciplines in order to learn how to use an interdisciplinary approach. Howard, Beauchesne, Shea, & Meservey (1997) found that faculty in medicine and nursing do not value interdisciplinary teaming as much as they value the maintenance of professional identity, perhaps because they do not know how to teach interdisciplinary care. Students and faculty alike view themselves according to traditional roles. Howard et al. (1997) advocate that students must be provided real experiences in which several disciplines work together in solving patient-care problems. Linking students with mentors who are involved in interdisciplinary practice is effective. Another helpful strategy is involving different groups of students in a community service initiative, for example, detecting and eliminating lead poisoning. The challenges of interdisciplinary education must be met if we are to truly achieve an integrated health care delivery system.

Summary

The blueprint for the future of health care is still being drawn. Health care organizations should seize every opportunity to plan their future. When all providers are committed to working within an integrated system, they can capitalize on their expertise in managing risks. When Nightingale's vision of ministering to whole beings becomes paramount in importance, all health care providers will accept the responsibility to serve clients well in an environment that promotes healing. By working together in a collaborative, consistent manner, health care providers can improve the health status of the community while still satisfying private and government purchasers of health care.

REFERENCES

Howard, E. P., Beauchesne, M. A., Shea, C. A., and Meservey, P. M. (1997). Research practicum: Linking education to practice. *Nurse Educator, 21,* 33–37.

Lasker, R. D. (1997). *Medicine and public health: The power of collaboration* (rev ed.). New York: New York Academy of Medicine.

Nightingale, F. (1860). *Notes on nursing.* London: Harrison and Sons.

Senge, P. M. (1990). The fifth discipline: The art and practice of the learning organization. New York: Doubleday Currency.

U.S. Department of Health and Human Services. (1997). Developing objectives for healthy people 2010. Washington, D.C.: Health and Human Services, Office of Disease Prevention and Health Promotion.

CHAPTER

2 Models for Building Healthy Communities

ANNETTE J. McBETH
KATHRYN D. SCHWEER

Our ability to create the future now will change behavior and thinking in the present.

—Dr. Moshe Rubinstein

- Community Primary Health Care Model
- Interactive Planning Process
- Considerations for Using the Interactive Planning Process
- Summary

The goal of healthy people and healthy communities was first established in 1979 by the report *Healthy People: The Surgeon General's Report on Health Promotion and Disease Prevention.* Throughout the country, communities found ways to achieve the goals of reducing mortality and increasing independent healthy lifestyles.

Research on health promotion and disease prevention expanded, and new objectives evolved into the next report, entitled *Healthy People 2000: National Health Promotion and Disease Prevention Objectives.* The three broad approaches of health promotion, health protection, and preventive services provided the framework for individuals to assess and modify their personal health behaviors, and for communities to evaluate their population's health.

Development of objectives for the first decade of the twenty-first century has been based on experiences of users and the changing context of health care. According to the resource guide *Developing Objectives for Healthy People 2010* (U.S. Department of Health and Human Services, 1997):

> Advances in preventive therapies, vaccines and pharmaceuticals, assistive technologies, and computerized systems will all change the face of medicine and how it is practiced. New relationships will be defined between public health departments and health care delivery organizations. Meanwhile, demographic changes in the United States—reflecting an older and more racially diverse population—will create new demands on public health and the overall health care system. Global forces—including food supplies, emerging infectious diseases, and environmental interdependence—will present new public health challenges. (p. 5)

The proposed framework for health in 2010 is presented in Figure 2.1. The goals for the nation of increasing years of healthy life and eliminating health disparities are to be achieved by four enabling goals: (1) promote healthy behaviors, (2) protect health, (3) assure access to quality health care, and (4) strengthen community prevention. Population-based activities that promote the health of individuals and communities are an important part of the framework.

Community Primary Health Care Model

The community primary health care model advocated in this chapter is based on the definition of primary health care set forth by the World Health Organization in 1978. According to this definition, primary health care is

> essential health care based on practical, scientifically sound and socially acceptable methods and technology made universally accessible to individuals and families in the community through their full participation and at a cost that the community and country can afford to maintain at every stage of their development in the spirit of self-reliance and self-determination. It forms an integral part both of the country's health system, of which it is the central function and main focus, and part of the overall social and economic development of the community. (World Health Organization, 1978)

The framework for the community primary health care model is built on community need and choice. The model provides an approach for constructing interventions that improve health outcomes. It embodies five principles (World Health Organization, 1978):

- Equitable distribution
- Appropriate technology
- A focus on health promotion and disease prevention
- Community participation
- A multisectorial approach

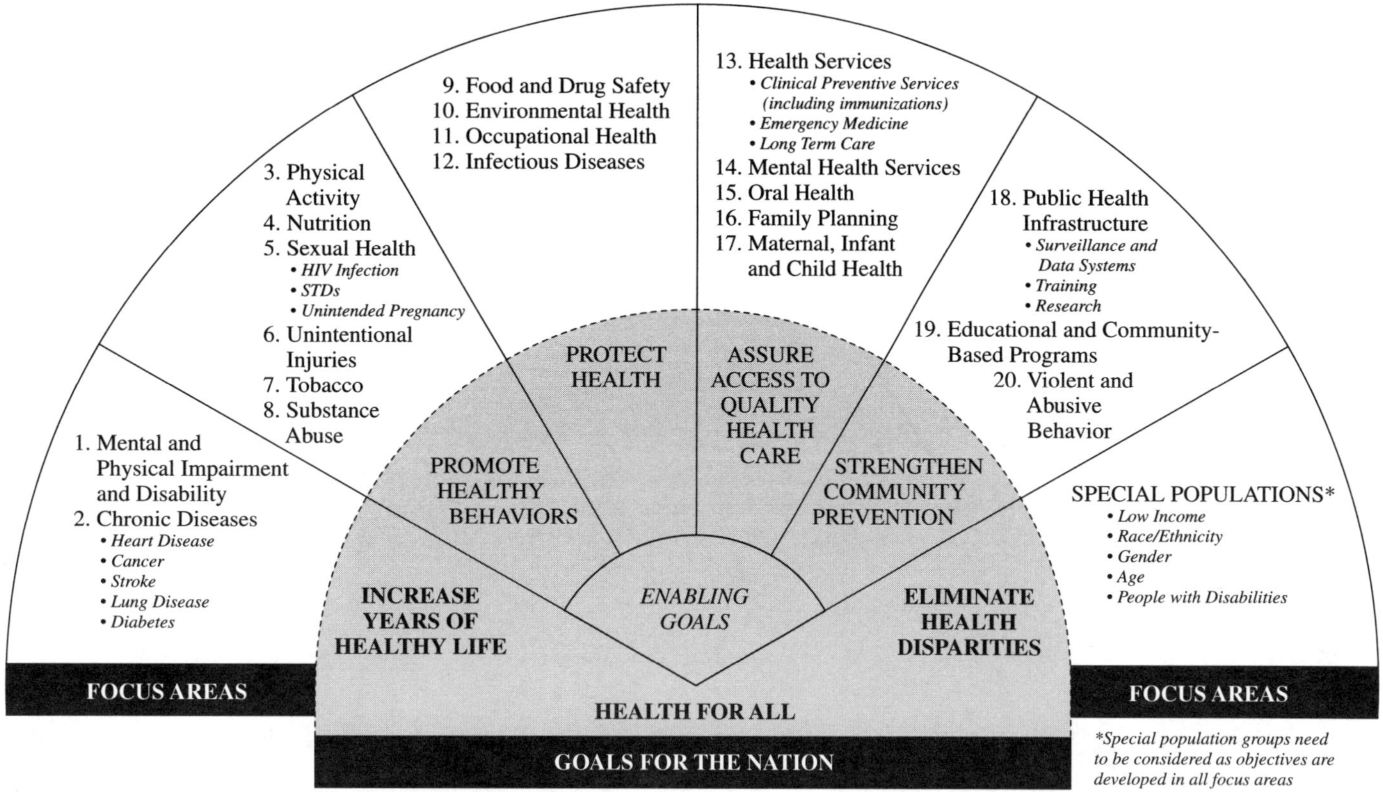

9. Food and Drug Safety
10. Environmental Health
11. Occupational Health
12. Infectious Diseases
13. Health Services
• Clinical Preventive Services (including immunizations)
• Emergency Medicine
• Long Term Care
14. Mental Health Services
15. Oral Health
16. Family Planning
17. Maternal, Infant and Child Health
3. Physical Activity
4. Nutrition
5. Sexual Health
• HIV Infection
• STDs
• Unintended Pregnancy
6. Unintentional Injuries
7. Tobacco
8. Substance Abuse
18. Public Health Infrastructure
• Surveillance and Data Systems
• Training
• Research
19. Educational and Community-Based Programs
20. Violent and Abusive Behavior
1. Mental and Physical Impairment and Disability
2. Chronic Diseases
• Heart Disease
• Cancer
• Stroke
• Lung Disease
• Diabetes
SPECIAL POPULATIONS*
• Low Income
• Race/Ethnicity
• Gender
• Age
• People with Disabilities
PROTECT HEALTH
ASSURE ACCESS TO QUALITY HEALTH CARE
PROMOTE HEALTHY BEHAVIORS
STRENGTHEN COMMUNITY PREVENTION
ENABLING GOALS
INCREASE YEARS OF HEALTHY LIFE
ELIMINATE HEALTH DISPARITIES
HEALTH FOR ALL
FOCUS AREAS
FOCUS AREAS
GOALS FOR THE NATION
*Special population groups need to be considered as objectives are developed in all focus areas

FIGURE 2.1 Vision of 2010: Healthy People in Healthy Communities

Source: From *Developing Objectives for Healthy People 2010.* Washington, D.C., Department of Health and Human Services, Office of Disease Prevention and Health Promotion, 1997.

Equitable distribution reflects the goal espoused in *Developing Objectives for Healthy People 2010* of eliminating health disparities. Segments of the population with specific health needs or special problems related to income, race, gender, age, or disabilities must be recognized. The entire community has a responsibility to help individuals in these groups receive the primary health care they need in order to achieve their full potential.

Appropriate technology includes an integrated information infrastructure, diagnostic and treatment modalities, transportation, communication networks, and other existing and emerging technologies. These technologies are tools communities use to assess their needs, provide interventions, and evaluate outcomes in relation to established goals of health for all.

A focus on health promotion and disease prevention includes not only primary care focused on personal health services and individual health behaviors, but also the development of health policies and prevention of diseases for all people. It seeks to uncover factors related to complex health problems so that prevention strategies can be explored.

Community participation is essential for building healthy communities. Health care providers must go beyond an interdisciplinary approach and become partners with community members. Risk-takers who have new visions of the goals of healthy communities, as well as their roles in achieving the goals, will be needed to participate in building healthy communities.

A multisectorial approach recognizes that the collaborative efforts in many sectors influence the health of all. Figure 2.2 illustrates a primary health care model that uses a multisectorial approach. The six major sectors in the model are interconnected. An event in one sector affects all other sectors positively or negatively and has an effect upon health for all.

A process that has proven effective for implementing the community primary health care model is the interactive planning process. All the principles of the model, especially the principles of community participation and a multisectorial approach, are incorporated into the interactive planning process.

Interactive Planning Process

Interactive planning is a process for creating and managing change in complex social systems and is based on two essential concepts: systems thinking and design (Ackoff, 1986; Ackoff, 1989).

Systems thinking is a way of defining problems in organizations. Complex social systems can be understood only through an analysis of the actions of their subparts. Hospitals and educational institutions are complex social systems with personnel, clients, and services that constantly act and interact. A community health care system is even more complex.

Design is a way of finding solutions and consists of cycles of imaging, presenting, and testing. Interactive planning participants share their own particular visions

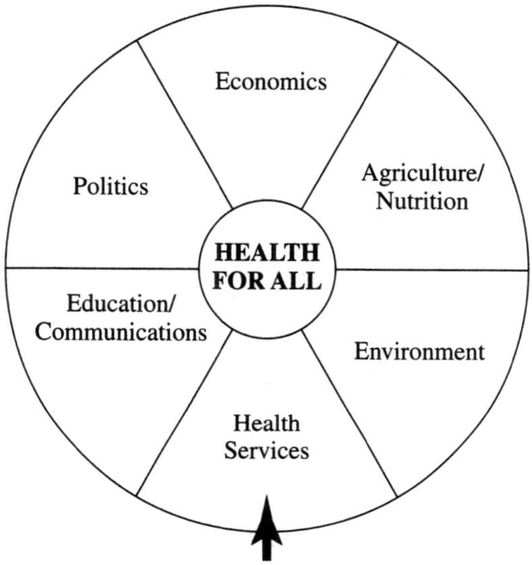

FIGURE 2.2 Primary Health Care Model

Source: Permission to reprint from Shoultz, J. and Hatcher, P. A. (1997). Looking beyond primary care to primary health care: An approach to community-based action, *Nursing Outlook, 45:* 23–25.

and discover common themes. In this way, members of the system develop a shared image and understanding. Testing is then done through action and evaluation. The process of interactive planning involves people at all levels, both inside and outside an organization. Interactive planning empowers those who participate. It demonstrates that change is possible at the individual level, group level, organizational level, and systems level. Eventually, change also will occur at the levels of the community and region.

Health care providers and community partners can use the interactive planning process with its systems thinking, design, and guiding principles to continuously improve the coordination of health care services both locally and regionally. Teams should be interdisciplinary as well as intra- and inter-organizational.

Considerations for Using the Interactive Planning Process

Education and training in the use of the interactive planning process will enable a community to design and build its own vision for a healthy community. The work of Russell Ackoff provides an excellent foundation for this process (Ackoff, 1986;

Ackoff, 1989). As described in Chapter 4, Creating a Shared Vision for a Healthy Community, it is essential to allow time for learning the process. As new community members become involved, they need to be oriented to the interactive planning process. Dedicated resources and commitment to the process need to be ensured.

Several principles guide the interactive planning process: planning backward, participation by all affected, continuous review of assumptions and expectations, and coordination and integration. The five phases of an interactive planning process include:

- Formulating the mess—defining current reality as seen by key stakeholders
- Ends planning—shared visioning of the future, with consensus on goals or ends to be attained
- Means planning—innovation in methods, procedures, and organization of efforts
- Resource planning—obtaining what you need in terms of funding, staffing, materials, and other resources
- Implementation—coordinating and sharing responsibility, authority, and accountability throughout the process.

Listed below are some steps which facilitate the use of the interactive planning process. The list is not exhaustive, but is intended to provide some guidance on how to develop the collaborative approach necessary for building healthy communities:

Principles

Planning backward

- Develop a shared vision utilizing the general themes of a cross section of the community
- Have each party describe the shared vision (e.g., what does *premier* or *best* mean to you?)
- Ask what each person's job would be like if the shared vision were realized
- Ask what each person would need to work this way (e.g., training, equipment, policies)
- Ask how these can be put in place and what is needed to make each step possible.

Participation by all affected

- Determine who interacts with the client and who provides direct or indirect services
- Consider family, friends, agencies, clergy, community resources, payers—in short, all who are affected
- Involve a cross section of diverse groups who will be affected.

Continuous review of assumptions and expectations

- Determine whether or not everyone understands the shared vision and if all newcomers agree with the shared vision

- Ask if expectations regarding changes to be made are clear to all involved (time lines, position descriptions, guidelines, policies)
- Ask what the assumptions are

Coordination and integration

- Check regularly with those above and below in organizational and community hierarchies
- Hold interactive discussions to see how changes are progressing
- Share plans before they are implemented, and utilize feedback to modify plans as appropriate
- Evaluate on an ongoing basis whether the vision is being achieved.

Phases

Formulating the mess

- Identify key stakeholders representing a cross section of the community
- Bring stakeholders together to ask for their perceptions of current reality
- Ask participants to respond to statements such as:

—I get frustrated when…
—The major cause of stress where I work is…
—We have to do a better job of…
—The complaint I hear most often is…
—Our major problem is…

- Analyze comments to determine recurrent themes of current reality
- Paint a word picture of primary health care in the community, and obtain reactions; use those reactions to expand the description of current reality
- Identify the gaps that exist in your setting and community
- Listen. Don't challenge. Perception is reality. Ask participants how experiences affected them, what they did about it, whom they told, what responses they received, and so on.

Ends planning

- Brainstorm ideas of what a healthy community would be like
- Develop consensus regarding important and essential outcomes—that is, your shared vision
- Identify goals based on community needs and establish priorities
- Establish a template for community care in the year 2010, setting goals which include:
  —Community needs
  —Populations served
  —Measurement targets

—Action steps that address
- what is to be measured
- who will collect the data
- who will provide the services
- where results will be archived
- benchmarks
- time lines

Means planning

- Ask what needs to change and determine what methods, policies, procedures, forms, etc., can be handled differently
- Determine if there is a better, easier, more cost-effective way to get the job done
- Find out if the leaders and staff are empowered to make things happen

Resource planning

- Determine what resources (money, time, people, materials, information, equipment, etc.) are needed
- Ask what needs to change to make the resources available
- Find out who controls the resources and whether they share the organization's vision

Implementation

- Clearly define and communicate the responsibility, authority, and accountability of every person involved
- Quickly communicate changes in the vision, plan, or schedules to all involved
- Regularly remind participants about systems thinking, the shared vision, implementation goals, and the overall design for achieving the shared vision
- Appoint a community-based steering committee representative of the key stakeholders to implement a community care 2010 plan

Summary

The World Health Organization and the United States Public Health Service have set forth goals for improving the health of people and communities. In order to achieve the goal of "health for all," a community primary health care model must be established and implemented. Principles of primary health care identified by the World Health Organization (1978) should underscore efforts to achieve the health goals of the nation.

How can people go about achieving healthy communities? A willingness to participate in new ways, a shared vision of what a healthy community would be like in a particular setting, and expanding the boundaries of concern are all important. A process for achieving these goals, the interactive planning process, can be implemented in many ways. Some suggestions for implementation have been presented for community groups to consider as they conduct the important work of building healthy communities.

Interactive planning and collaboration are invaluable strategies for focusing on the health needs of communities, the nation, and the world. They offer hope to an otherwise dismal prospect. The resources, both human and fiscal, exist when communities become health focused and can work together in an integrated system based on common values and a common vision.

REFERENCES

Ackoff, R. L. (1989). Executive summaries—The circular organization: An update. *Academy of Management Executives, 3,* 11–16.

Ackoff, R. L. (1986). *Management in small doses.* New York: John Wiley & Sons.

Healthy People: The Surgeon General's report on health promotion and disease prevention. (1979). Department of Health, Education, and Welfare, Public Health Service, Washington, D.C.

Rubinstein, M. (1998). *Backward thinking: Embracing uncertainty and chaos and thriving; An agenda for the future.* American Association of Colleges of Nursing Summer Seminar. Leadership in the Face of Change: Lessons from Industry. Seattle, WA: July 26–29, 1998.

Shoultz, J. & Hatcher, P. A. (1997). Looking beyond primary care to primary health care: An approach to community-based action. *Nursing Outlook, 1997,* 23–26.

U.S. Department of Health and Human Services. (1997). Developing objectives for healthy people 2010. Washington, D.C.: Department of Health and Human Services, Office of Disease Prevention and Health Promotion.

World Health Organization. (1978). Primary health care: Report of the International Conference on Primary Health Care. Geneva, Switzerland: World Health Organization.

CHAPTER

3 Regionalization

KRISTIN JULIAR

DOUGLAS L. WOOD

ANNETTE J. McBETH

We must build a new world, a far better world—one in which the eternal dignity of man is respected.

—Harry Truman

- Forces Challenging Health Care
  - —Social Forces
  - —Political Forces
  - —Economic Forces
  - —Technological Forces
- Key Components of Regionalization
  - —Shared Decision Making and Governance
  - —Regional Health Care Planning
  - —Population-Based Approach
- Health Promotion and Disease Prevention
- The Power of the Consumer
- Major Concepts of Regionalization
- Summary

Regionalization as an organizational model for health care has many proponents. This model has recently been found to be ideal in the context of controlling health care costs, meeting the needs of primary health care, preventing diseases, and promoting healthy lifestyles.

In the twenty-first century, health care will have to become organized on a systematic regional basis. Indeed, some providers have already moved to a national or international focus as their systems have grown. Within a regional system, the focus should be on providing an integrated system to improve the health status of its people and communities. This will involve new affiliations among people and agencies that have not worked together in the past. The resources and skills of provider groups, institutions, government, community organizations, and educational units can then achieve a higher level of functioning through collaboration.

Many social, political, economic, and technical forces are having a profound effect on the health of people in our society. The health care industry will need to create partnerships in order to meet the challenges of these societal forces. The development of partnerships between providers and institutions, together with partnerships between public and private entities, will help address regional needs cost-effectively.

In the twenty-first century, organizations must leave turf issues behind and focus on community and regional needs to achieve identified goals for a healthy region and nation. Individuals and organizations must join forces with policymakers on the local, state, and national level to address societal health issues. For example, while stop smoking programs may help individuals, policies that reduce juvenile access to tobacco products and tobacco subsidies, restrictions on tobacco advertising, and other laws will have a greater effect on society (U.S. Department of Health and Human Services, 1995). *Healthy People 2010* outlines the framework for achieving health goals for the nation (see Chapter 2, Figure 2.1). Regional efforts must ensure consumer choices for acute and chronic health care, as well as implementation of health promotion guidelines and disease prevention services. Shared decision making and partnerships will be important in regional health planning. The consumer will be the ultimate judge and should be a principal partner in the planning and implementation processes. As the consumer makes choices in health care, regional outcomes will be evaluated for accessibility, affordability, availability, and acceptability.

Forces Challenging Health Care

Several forces outside the health care delivery system affect the health of communities. In American society, changes in family life have contributed to unhealthy behaviors. Political forces have altered people's perspectives about the role of government in providing health care services. Pressures to control costs have changed relationships between consumers and providers. Major technological advances have changed most aspects of health care delivery. These forces are described in further detail.

Social Forces

In a disease-focused health care system, crime and violence are often perceived as an emergency room issue. In fact, violence accounts for millions of dollars of health care costs and unnecessary absenteeism in the workplace. In a more systematic and community-oriented approach, crime and violence can be envisioned as a health care issue that affects all populations, but especially children, women, the elderly, and those with lower incomes. Crime and violence can also be viewed in terms of community needs for education, job availability, and retraining in order to secure a safe environment for individuals and their families. Therefore, health care providers and payers, along with community stakeholders, must work together to find ways to reduce social isolation and prevent crime and violence. Such efforts might include devoting money to education, housing, and economic development rather than to expensive emergency room care, long-term care, or welfare payments for those unable to work because of injuries suffered in violent acts.

Health care professionals educated in traditional programs might not immediately understand their role in addressing social problems. Public health activities provided through local and state governments often operate parallel and separate from private health care systems. This happens because health care systems focus on disease and individuals, while public health focuses on the overall health of the community. Community-based organizations are increasingly adopting a public health approach to address specific community needs, such as violence, substance abuse, child abuse, or care of the elderly.

It is critical for these three systems—private health care, governmental public health, and community-based organizations—to link efforts in a regional approach to address such community needs. One area to explore is the role of health care professionals in addressing crime and violence. Since crime and violence interfere with good health, it is important to identify the health promotion and prevention efforts that could be implemented to reduce crime and violence in our communities (U.S. Department of Health and Human Services, 1997a). Efforts aimed at identifying family situations where there is a potential for violence could help reduce the utilization of emergency and other medical resources to treat injuries as well as to improve the social functioning of individuals and families. Efforts at removing firearms from the home would reduce the potential for injury and the incidence of teen suicide. Educational efforts in the elementary and secondary schools aimed at conflict resolution and avoidance of drugs would save lives and avoid injuries. Health screening practices could identify crime and violence as factors in a patient's life and health. Incorporating risk assessment questions as part of an annual review of lifestyle practices could be an easily undertaken and effective method to identify opportunities for intervention.

A second area involves the way in which private health professionals address child abuse and neglect in the community. There are ways to identify potential neglect and to intervene before the child is harmed. Efforts aimed at determining risk factors in family situations could result in identification of families needing support during the prenatal period. For example, public health and/or maternal child health nurses and volunteers could make regular home visits to provide support, advice, and encouragement to the parents. As parenting skills develop, the risk of child abuse decreases.

As this thinking evolves, health professionals will learn to be a part of the population- and community-based approach to reducing and preventing crime and violence. This cannot happen effectively in isolation. For example, if a hospital starts a campaign to reduce violence and shoulders all the work, the campaign can expect to have limited effectiveness. If, however, the hospital joins with other community organizations, such as schools, churches, law enforcement, social services, public health, youth organizations, senior citizen groups, and poverty organizations, it can bring its special expertise and resources to bear in a comprehensive approach that uses the resources of these other groups. The hospital will, in turn, learn from its involvement with the community and be better prepared to identify abuse, provide referrals for those who have been abused, share resources to prevent child abuse or protect homebound elderly from caregiver abuse, and try other community approaches with potential for success. The importance of conducting a united effort is evident from mortality statistics. Homicide is the number-two reason for mortality for adolescents and number fourteen for the total population (U.S. Department of Health and Human Services, 1997b).

As with crime and violence, other social problems can be understood as health issues. These include poverty and welfare dependence, substance abuse, and poor family functioning. Again, the opportunities to develop a potent and effective integrated system are significant.

The health care system can approach the consequences of social issues on a case by case basis, or it can join with community organizations to address these issues. Following are two examples that demonstrate the need for a community approach.

A widow dependent on Social Security is admitted to a hospital, malnourished and dehydrated. There are signs that she has been physically abused. She is fed and rehydrated, and her wounds are tended. What role can the hospital take in assuring that she will not later return to the hospital in the same condition? What services are available to protect her from further abuse? How can the hospital work with community organizations to expand senior nutrition programs? How can the health care system join forces with community organizations to prevent elder abuse? The development of community-based interventions, perhaps using volunteers who make frequent visits to elderly persons, can help identify the need for social and other support services. Referrals to and follow-up by home health care nurses would be appropriate in the case described above. Nutrition services, caregiver support, and other community-based services may be needed to achieve the goal of prevention of elder abuse. Can formal linkages with public health, aging programs, and community organizations be created?

The second example involves the case of an infant born with fetal alcohol syndrome, which results in serious, permanent, yet entirely preventable birth defects. Can community groups use the schools, colleges, media, and public information campaigns to promote prevention? Can obstetricians, midwives, and other primary care providers perform a major role in prevention by thoroughly screening for alcohol consumption and abuse in patient interviews? Can they then provide education and support, or refer patients to appropriate community resources? Can health care organizations or systems create treatment programs specifically targeted toward women with children? The combined efforts of health care providers and community groups could create a safety net for pregnant women and women of child-bearing age. The outcome could be reduced substance use during pregnancy.

Systems thinking of this type helps define the role of the health care industry in addressing key social problems. By viewing itself as a subset of the larger community and working in partnership with other community organizations and institutions, the health care industry will be better able to address social problems that affect it.

Political Forces

Although local and state health departments have made major contributions to community health through public hygiene and sanitation measures, disease control, health assessment, policy development, and regulations, an integrated community-based health system has not been developed. Current health care systems do not always focus on consumer needs and fail to provide a continuum of care. Although some members of the community may have access to all the health care services they need, others are denied access to basic services.

Integrated planning is required at the state, regional, and national level. Government is challenged to keep up with rapid changes in the health care industry. While government commands enormous resources to pay for health services, limited resources are available for health promotion, care of populations with special needs, and health education programs. Future limitations on the ability to cover the costs of such programs from tax revenues will limit the resources available to predict, shape, and lead change in the health care industry.

Currently, federal Medicare and Medicaid dollars are allocated to the states. Some states are distributing these resources to regional empowerment zones. Herein lies an opportunity to become architects of healthy communities for the future. Shifting the ways in which financial resources become available would allow communities to

- Hire or seek consultation with the best health care policy administrators and thinkers. Many visionary people in government, academia, and private foundations are hired by private industry for much more money than is currently available in the government sector.
- Lobby for community-based perspectives in partnership with regional and national stakeholders.
- Convene regional coordinating boards to prepare the public for dramatic changes in the health care system, shifting the focus to healthy people, families, and communities.
- Assume leadership in addressing regional health issues in order to assure access to health care for all people.

State and national health care systems have become so complex that governments are hard-pressed to keep up with them. For example, state health departments cannot project their needs for health care professionals without first surveying major health systems in the state to determine their plans. Discrepancies that occur in recruitment and location of health care professionals as a result of multiple systems working separately to achieve strategic plans can be wasteful. Duplication of services in some areas and continued lack of adequate numbers of providers in other areas are a result of the current lack of collaboration and coordination.

To some degree, this discrepancy reflects the private distrust of government planning efforts and the potential limitations that may be imposed on private entities by the government. It would be advantageous for providers in a region to undertake collaborative needs assessments and planning to improve the health of individuals, families, and communities. However, such activities have been viewed by government as anticompetitive and subject to antitrust laws. Careful work among legislatures, the executive branch of federal and state governments, and health care providers will be necessary to overcome the barriers to systems thinking and success that are currently legislated. Public health agencies can collaborate with managed care organizations around public health goals. Collaboration between the public and private sectors will be essential to meet this challenge and to assure that underserved and high-risk groups will be effectively served in the future.

At the local level, a paradox exists: universal unwillingness to accept any change in the established delivery systems and a belief in the ability to plan and carry out any state or national changes locally. If the state and nation are ill-equipped to plan and manage the profound changes in the health care system, communities are even more handicapped. Few local elected officials see any role beyond attempting to preserve the services they currently offer. Few private providers and institutions see any role beyond preserving or enhancing their position in the market and their financial position. This can change only when communities envision themselves as a client base and work as partners with health provider systems to develop health services addressing the unique needs of the community (Amundson, 1993). For example, the communities of Chisago City, Rush City, and Forest Lake in Minnesota have demonstrated the effectiveness of such approaches. Each of these small communities decided that acute care inpatient hospital services should no longer be available in each community but that instead a new regional hospital should be designed and built to meet the needs of the entire region. The existing hospital buildings were then reconfigured to more effectively support primary care practices in each city. The result has been growth in the number of providers of care within the region, rather than the loss of providers many predicted. Though this change was facilitated by the involvement of a single health care system, each community, each medical staff, and each hospital staff had to reach a consensus to support such a regional plan (Amundson, 1993).

Economic Forces

Who controls the money spent on health care? Even in an impoverished rural community, millions of dollars are spent annually on health care. Where do these dollars go? The more of those dollars a community captures, the greater the benefit to the overall economy of the area (Amundson, 1993).

As the twentieth century comes to a close, limited resources at all levels have placed the focus on management of costs and resources. Payers have become major decision makers in health care. When payers are looking at overall costs to the system, the decision making changes dramatically. Efforts at managing costs have included limiting care options (e.g., coverage for minor problems, such as ear infections) and finding methods of reducing costs within a system (e.g., downsizing or restructuring). Rohrer indicates that

> the community health system cannot exist independently of the larger health care system in which it is embedded. Local systems need big partners from whom they can acquire technical expertise and other resources; and with whom they can share financial risk. (Rohrer, 1996, p. 37)

If costs within the system are to be reduced, then there must be some method of managing and coordinating all processes within the system in order to improve efficiency and quality. Regionalization will allow a more systematic approach to managing the system by being stewards of available resources. Each institution need not be a complete health care system in and of itself, like most community hospitals were in the past. Through integrated regionalization, institutions can specialize in primary care or various specialties, and share their resources. Additional savings can be accomplished through regional integration of fixed costs in administrative, information, and clinical services, among other areas. Community-based organizations can join with health care systems to achieve local health improvement goals.

Technological Forces

Technology both creates and reduces costs. Technological advances are keeping patients alive at a high cost, both for the interventions using technology and for the added chronic care costs incurred for survivors of previously fatal illnesses. Networks providing regional linkages will be the norm as we enter the twenty-first century. Telemedicine, teleradiology, and telecommunications allow specialty services at remote locations. For example, rather than having patients from rural areas travel to urban medical centers for consultation, doctors use telemedicine to consult with them at neighborhood clinics or hospitals. Where this model is in place, patients have the resources of the larger, specialized hospital without spending time and money traveling long distances.

Telecommunications have potential for in-home care as well, especially for chronically ill patients with limited mobility. The difficulty of transporting frail elderly or chronically ill individuals may result in nursing home placements to avoid the problems and inconveniences of transfers from home to physician office. However, when home care nurses consult with the physician by telemedicine, frail persons remain in their homes longer. In-home telecommunication links to monitor compliance and provide frequent patient interaction will result in better care for patients with chronic illness, including fewer hospital admissions and shorter hospital stays.

Telecommunications are also having a profound effect on emergency care. Computer linkages allow emergency medical technicians (EMTs) to consult about protocols and to interact in a sophisticated manner with the emergency service facility in order to implement life-saving measures on site. Real-time information from the site of the emergency or from a smaller hospital that has stabilized a patient prior to transfer to a trauma center allows the receiving team to be fully prepared when the patient arrives. This coordination is especially valuable when distance and long response times would otherwise threaten the survival of the patient.

Television and Internet access are changing how people gather health care information. Education channels on television broadcast demonstrations of surgical procedures, reports on the latest health-related research, and a variety of health promotion information. Internet users can find accurate and timely information on health conditions, health providers, health insurers, and health care options. They will also expect to receive health care services, to schedule appointments, and to order products electronically. Information technology allows resources located virtually anywhere to be utilized elsewhere. Dispatching for emergency medical service, for example, can now occur anywhere. Medical students in residency in isolated clinics and hospitals can link with their schools for library materials, consultation classes, and interaction with their peers. Disease management strategies and best-practice guidelines can be incorporated into intranet (or Internet) applications to improve the quality of care delivered by physicians and other providers. Computer applications can also enhance the ability of physicians to understand the consequences of their actions by entering their data into databases with statistical analysis and reporting capabilities. Another application of information technology is a population-based immunization registry, which could be accessed by all health care providers in the region. Distance education links educational resources to local needs for health care workforce development and continuing education.

A regional approach to using technological advances in patient care is also needed. The certificate-of-need process for authorizing large-scale, high-cost technology, such as CAT scanners or neonatal intensive care services, has not universally contained costs. Regional collaboration and cooperation will be essential in removing waste and duplication while still making these technologies available to the public. Such collaboration may involve consolidation of provider groups or development of partnerships between hospitals and physicians. It will be necessary to remove legal constraints that make joint ventures difficult to arrange. New and better measures of performance need to be developed, so that providers will be able to demonstrate that their actions are responsible in both fiduciary and community service dimensions. Decisions about acquisition and implementation of new technology should be made only after a careful consideration of the needs of the community and the development of a technology plan that will permit the most effective use of dollars.

Key Components of Regionalization

Hospitals and other health care institutions were established to serve community needs. As their expertise in illness care developed, people from outside the community turned to these institutions for care. Traditionally, hospitals have added new technology and services without systematic assessment of the health care needs of the region.

A hospital is often a health care leader in a community. The community benefits when the hospital shares leadership with other health care organizations. Nord describes the outcomes of such a partnership in Laramie, Wyoming:

> The measurable benefit from this community partnership is evident: a new service for the community. The less tangible benefit from this alliance is improved communication, accurate information and a spirit of cooperation that is remarkable in today's competitive society. (Nord, 1993, p. 19)

In order to offer regional health care services efficiently and effectively, local and state governments, health care organizations, agencies, and consumers of health care must be involved in collaborative planning. City, county, state, and national boundaries will have less relevance in the twenty-first century. A region may instead be defined on the basis of shared problems, needs, and resources. Successful approaches will utilize a broad population base. Regionalization of both health promotion and disease prevention services will be required. As a result, natural regional systems will evolve with strategically integrated health centers that are easily accessible.

Shared Decision Making and Governance

Successful regionalization depends on shared decision making and governance. Hierarchical models and organizational charts do a poor job of delineating responsibilities and levels of interaction. Circular models, which utilize spheres of responsibility and defined areas of collaborating, and identify where joint decision making occurs, are more useful for endeavors of regionalization.

Figure 3.1 is an organizational chart that demonstrates a regional partnership. Each point is composed of several agencies, organizations, and/or businesses. An agency, organization, or business that has more than one purpose can appear in more than one of the points. For example, a hospital could be a provider network, or a service-education partner, or a member of the technology council.

A specific example of a regional community care partnership can be found in south-central Minnesota. The Region Nine Community Care Partnership's organizational chart, shown in Figure 3.2, links the work of the individual funding partners in the areas of common interest and concern. This work has been supported by matching funds from The Robert Wood Johnson Foundation Local Initiatives Funding Partners Program. Representatives from each of the funding partners meet with the

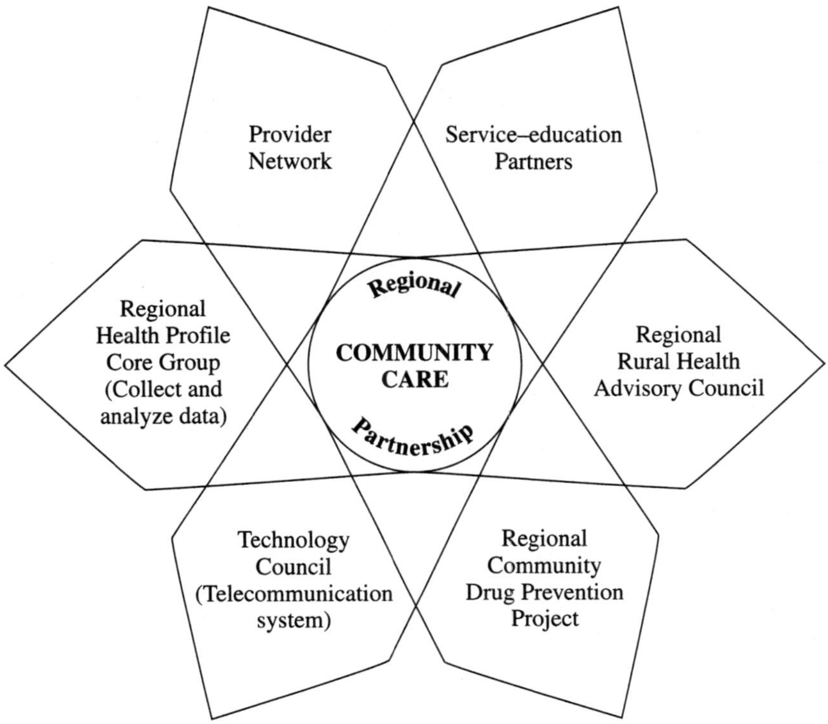

FIGURE 3.1 Regional Community Care Partnership

Source: From material developed by Anne Ganey, Project Director, Region Nine Community Care Partnership (1999). By permission.

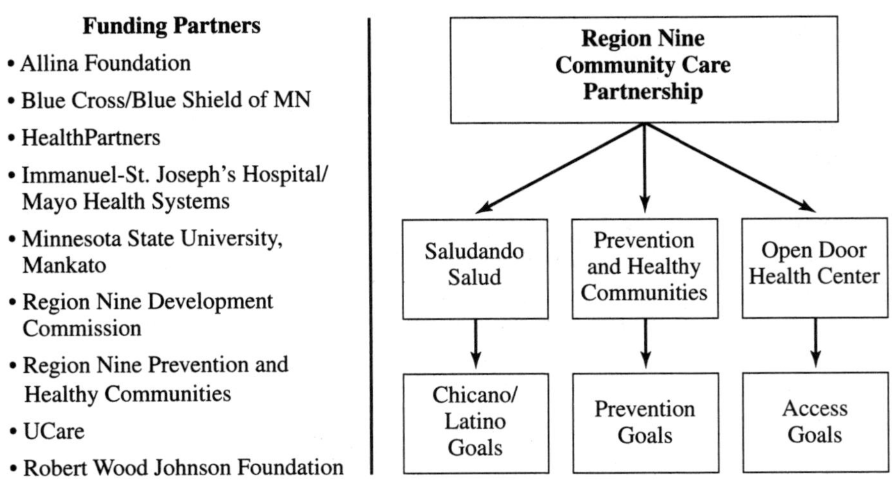

FIGURE 3.2 Region Nine Community Care Partnership

Source: From material developed by Anne Ganey, Project Director, Region Nine Community Care Partnership (1999). By permission.

partnership to address common goals. At the same time, each individual partner continues its own work.

Partnership members work together to create a collaborative model across competitors, acting as a community voice in shaping the evolving system. Thus far, the partnership has

- Established the Open Door Health Center, which serves the uninsured and underinsured
- Conducted two regional health profiles
- Begun integration of a management information system into a single data repository, from which data will be shared regionally across public and private organizations
- Developed a community service plan that focuses on healthy infants and youth, healthy families, aging populations, and access and affordability of health care
- Implemented a health outreach program for Chicano/Latino residents

These examples demonstrate that a regional, population-based approach focused on community needs can be successful. Health care professionals can be highly resistant to community involvement in health care decision making and governance. Strong leadership from primary health care providers is critical to success in regionalization (Satinsky, 1998).

Health care is changing, and much of the change is being driven by consumers, payers, and purchasers. Health care providers and professional organizations may resist changes proposed by those outside the health care system. Feeling under attack, they may cling to their role as the experts in health care. But the public seeks a new approach. Health care providers must recognize that, while they are experts in diagnosis and treatment of disease, patients and purchasers have much to say about health care accessibility, affordability, and acceptability. The recent rapid change in health care has created an erosion of trust among physicians, patients, purchasers, and payers.

Opening the doors to community involvement requires new partnerships between health providers and consumers. This does not diminish the expertise of health professionals, nor diminish their role in providing health services. In this model, health care professionals are necessary, but not sufficient, sources of expertise. The other experts needed reside in the community; they include citizens, educators, clergy, volunteers, government officials, and community organization volunteers and staff. The combined efforts of all with interest in health care delivery will be needed to be successful and cost-effective in community and regional integration efforts.

The list of people who need to participate in improving patient care and community health will grow as the concept of regionalization becomes integrated into the health care system. All health care workers across the continuum of care, along with workers in nontraditional roles, will need to work with the patient and family in order to achieve optimal health care. Promoting family strengths and individual responsibility will be important. The health care industry must educate itself on (1) the contributions and availability of all health disciplines; (2) options and organizations available to the community for diagnosis and treatment of acute and chronic disease; (3) support for caregivers; (4) health promotion, including primary, secondary, and tertiary prevention; (5) health counseling; (6) health education; and (7) health information needs. Then it can begin to incorporate this knowledge into practice and teach the community.

An example of this synergism is the Saludando Salud Project: Saying Hello to Health (Region Nine Development Commission, 1996–1997). This project was designed to re-create a rural health system to accommodate the needs of a new large immigrant population of Hispanic residents. The project combines the resources of a regional healthy communities project, local health and human service providers, employers, public radio, bilingual residents, colleges, churches, and schools. Working together, they are training interpreters, retraining health professionals, providing community-based clinics, sponsoring a Spanish-language radio health call-in show, and providing outreach services. This project grew out of the realization by local health care providers that they lacked the expertise and resources to adequately provide health services to the new residents of their community. The health providers were willing to consult a variety of resources, including the new residents themselves. A community-based system has been developed by focusing very clearly on the health and culture of the Hispanic population; by using Hispanic interpreters, planners, and outreach workers; and by integrating health care services with other community resources.

Regional Health Care Planning

The ideal outcome of community planning on a regional basis would be ongoing active involvement by community members in designing future health care in their communities, working as partners with health care experts. No single entity can possibly provide all the health services needed by a community. Communities and regional health providers can articulate which services are best delivered in a community-based service model and which services need to be provided elsewhere or by other providers within the region. Creativity in integrating regional services with locally delivered community-based services will assure success.

An example illustrates the need for integration. An elderly stroke patient is about to be discharged from a tertiary care center to his home fifty miles away. What health care needs do this person and his family or support system have? What health care professional is planning the discharge? To whom does the caregiver(s) turn with questions? Who is helping them manage the recovery in the home? Who is helping to follow instructions from the tertiary care center? To whom will the caregiver(s) turn if the patient's condition deteriorates? Does the family or other caregiver(s) need home nursing or assistance with feeding and bathing the patient? How will they deal with the patient's depression? What resources are available to help them with financial problems resulting from the hospitalization and follow-up care? Which of these issues is dealt with through regional resources, and which through local providers? Who ties the two together? What personnel and technological connections would help the patient and the family or support system? Cases and questions like these can spark a regional effort to integrate services. None of these issues is biophysical, but rather the sequelae of a medical condition which cannot be addressed solely in a medical model.

The objectives for successful regional health care planning are to

- Engage a broad-based regional planning group of community members in identifying the critical health issues of the community
- Draw upon experts as a resource
- Assess the internal and external market forces
- Identify opportunities and threats related to the critical health issues delineated by the regional planning group
- Create linkages among health care and related services that focus needed resources on local health needs
- Design and implement strategies that bring local and outside resources together in a systematic approach to health care delivery that will meet the needs identified by the regional planning group
- Provide ongoing planning and technical assistance to communities
- Measure outcomes over a defined period of time

Population-Based Approach

Regionalization of health care services uses a population-based approach to identify health care needs. The region is analyzed in terms of health status, demographic characteristics, and geographic distribution, rather than by the location of the clinics and hospitals. Instead of looking at the number of health professionals employed relative to population density, an analysis of the availability of health professionals and services relative to the identified health care needs of the region is conducted.

For example, the Region Nine Community Care Partnership (1999) analyzed the population characteristics of the region and identified the following factors with implications for health care:

- An aging population disproportionately located in rural areas with few or no health care providers
- Volunteer emergency medical response systems in most communities
- Extremely high rates of poverty among single mothers with children under age six
- Numerous individuals engaged in hazardous occupations
- A large concentration of college-age individuals
- Difficulty in recruiting and retaining health care professionals and allied health professionals in small communities

The state's regional planning and development commission convened a community care partnership meeting consisting of private health care and public health providers, higher education institutions, and the major health systems and payers serving a nine-county area. This group identified joint health prevention and promotion priorities and is currently designing coordinated health promotion and prevention programs. An outcome of this community care partnership meeting was described above (see Figure 3.2).

Rural areas find it difficult to provide traditional health services because of limited financial and other resources. They have been forced to look for resources in the larger region and to combine these resources with a creative mix of local options. Some small communities have combined local health care facilities (hospital, clinic, nursing home) to share fixed costs. Others provide health services in community settings, such as schools, senior centers, or work sites. Parish nurses and rural hospice programs link volunteers with health professionals. Demand for hospital beds has diminished, and health care resources have been refocused on prevention, health promotion, convalescence, and home-based services. Other services are provided at regional centers.

Health Promotion and Disease Prevention

Health promotion and disease prevention services must be available at any point that care, support, or information is accessed. When health promotion and disease prevention are integrated into people's lives, the overall well-being of the community will improve. People will live longer, and the health of older persons will improve. Integrating health promotion and disease prevention will remove stress from some lives and will permit others to manage stress and ultimately enhance their quality of life.

A regional approach to addressing community health needs could include establishing coalitions to prevent substance abuse or teenage pregnancy. By combining resources, hospitals, public health agencies, educators, and planning agencies can conduct regional risk assessment surveys providing a profile, together with a data analysis of health promotion and disease prevention needs. This information can then be utilized to develop specific disease prevention and health promotion programs, such as DARE (Drug Abuse Resistance Education), use of bicycle helmets, diabetes screening, influenza immunizations, or approaches to secondary prevention of heart disease, stroke, or malignancy.

Addressing community and regional needs for health care delivery and health information requires an integrated approach. By involving the print and electronic media, resources of schools, churches, businesses, hospitals, public health agencies, clinics, and other community groups, an effective response can be achieved. Emphasis should be placed on the need for communities and individuals to be responsible for optimizing their own health potential and to decide how to use finite resources to care for individuals and for the community at large. Then, and only then, will the health of communities and people in the region be improved.

The Power of the Consumer

If regionalization is to take place in health care, stakeholders must be identified. The consumer is the key stakeholder. To provide quality care or a quality product, it is necessary to understand consumer desires and expectations. Services and products that exceed consumer expectations must be provided.

Changes in the delivery of health care may cause consumers to feel fear of the unknown or fear of being judged. These fears most often appear as anger, paranoia, or distrust. It is therefore vital to provide accurate and easily understood information and to involve consumers in health care decisions. In this manner, both the individual's and the community's ability to move forward and work collaboratively for the health of the community will be assured.

It is likewise important for trusting, effective working relationships to be established with payers. The payers will also have to understand their roles in integration of health care delivery and be willing to make financial commitments in different ways than have been customary in the past.

Consumers want community health care services to be accessible when needed and responsible to perceived needs. Services must be affordable and available at appropriate times. Since it is not possible to provide all services in all communities, it will be necessary to balance the availability of services against the cost of services, thus requiring a community decision about affordability. The responsibility for deciding which services are acceptable and affordable and how to make the services available and accessible rests on the community.

People are the experts about their own community. Outside experts can provide information, clarify discussion, and suggest potential solutions. Ultimately, however, community members are responsible for creating their own vision of a healthy community and for determining how to allocate scarce resources. They are the ones who know what the people of their community will accept.

People tend to focus on their own needs and the needs of their own organization. They feel threatened by change that disrupts their organization or lessens their control of resources. Yet a lessening of personal and organizational control is exactly what must happen to meet consumer and community needs, especially when consumer needs are in direct conflict with how an organization functions. For example, schools may not want parents to enter the building unless authorized. Employers may refuse to let health educators take employee time away from production. Designing an integrated, community-based system focused on consumer needs may be very difficult. True integration will require innovative approaches to developing solutions that effectively meet individual, local, and regional needs. Health care providers can play a valuable role in integrating separate services focused on individual needs. They can be partners, navigators, and role models not only to consumers but also to the organizations and communities they are serving.

Major Concepts of Regionalization

Health providers, community-based organizations, and governmental organizations can develop formal or informal collaborative organizations to collect and analyze data on health issues in the community. They can then go through a strategic planning effort to identify methods for each to work in concert at addressing these needs.

There must be representation in this process by individuals who have the knowledge to identify and analyze the effect of the health issues, and representation or strong support from top administrators who can allocate resources (staff, funds, and facilities) to implement the strategies.

Health providers and their community partners must aggressively seek roles on state and federal committees and commissions that develop policies with local impact. Organizations must budget staff time to travel to and participate in these policy efforts. Local groups should work together to identify legislative agendas that can be supported by a broad base of community organizations, health providers, and local governments. They must build relationships with their state and national elected officials and provide numerous opportunities for them to see what is going on in health care in the communities.

Leadership and education are critical. Leaders in health care and the community must introduce ideas for sharing costs, establishing relationships with other organizations, and restructuring organizations. Leaders must spend time educating the community, their boards, and potential collaborators about the long-term financial stability and quality of care that these changes will bring.

Community and population-based planning approaches are public health functions as well as functions of city, county, regional, and state planning agencies. Private health care facilities are frequently heavily engaged in marketing, strategic planning, and creating new visions for their organizations. Academic institutions are also engaged in planning. There is much value in bringing these different perspectives together. The first step is to convene a meeting to begin the process of joint planning. The meeting may be on a single health issue (e.g., drugs and underage drinking), or very broad in scope. Over time, these organizations can establish ongoing processes for joint planning around a variety of health issues, as well as the overall health of the region.

It is often easy to motivate public and private organizations to work together around specific health issues, such as teen pregnancy or immunization. As communities gain experience, joint planning will become the accepted way to deal with health issues as they arise. It will become an automatic response. Chapter 5 includes a description of a community-wide, coordinated, collaborative effort to address a meningitis outbreak in Mankato, Minnesota. Because the health and community organizations (hospital, clinics, public health, county government, schools, media, city, and nonprofit organizations) had been working together over a period of years on health and youth issues, there were strong relationships in place that allowed them to quickly respond to a disease outbreak in the community.

Community members will not take responsibility for addressing health issues unless they understand the role they play and the expertise they bring to the equation. For example, fetal alcohol syndrome can be prevented when professional health educators and social workers involve community members in speaking to community organizations, schools, families, and businesses on the hazards of alcohol use during pregnancy. The media can provide strong messages about the potential damage to the unborn child. Leadership is essential to both understand the role that community members can play and to articulate that role in a way that makes sense.

Summary

Regionalization of health care is both a challenge and an opportunity. A vision of healthy people and healthy communities will be the guide. When key stakeholders are involved in planning to meet the needs of the population, a focus on health promotion and disease prevention using a regional approach will emerge. Regional endeavors hold the best hope for building healthy communities.

REFERENCES

Amundson, B. (1993). Myth and reality in the rural health service crisis: Facing up to community responsibilities. *Journal of Rural Health, 9,* 176–187.

Bartlett, J. (1992). *Familiar Quotations: A collection of passages, phrases, and proverbs.* Boston: Little & Brown.

Nord, T. A. (1993). Ivinson Memorial Hospital, Laramie, WY.

Region Nine Development Commission. (1996–1997). *Saludando Salud quarterly report.* Washington, D.C.: Health Resources and Services Administration.

Region Nine Development Commission. (1999). *Region Nine Community Care Partnership.* Developed for The Robert Wood Johnson Foundation Local Initiatives Partnership Program grant, Mankato, MN.

Rohrer, J. E. (1996). *Planning for community-oriented health systems.* Washington, D.C.: American Public Health Association.

Satinsky, M. A. (1998). *The foundations of integrated care: Facing the challenges of change.* Chicago: American Hospital Publishing, Inc.

U.S. Department of Health and Human Services, Public Health Service. (1995). *Healthy people 2000: Midcourse review and 1995 revisions.* Sudbury, MA: Jones and Bartlett Publishers.

U.S. Department of Health and Human Services. (1997a). *Developing objectives for healthy people 2010.* Washington, D.C.: Health and Human Services, Office of Disease Prevention and Health Promotion.

U.S. Department of Health and Human Services. (1997b). *Morbidity and Mortality Weekly Reports.* Atlanta: Centers for Disease Control.

CHAPTER

4 Creating a Shared Vision for a Healthy Community

SHARON P. AADALEN
JEROME A. CREST
MARY I. HUNTLEY

Never doubt that a small group of thoughtful, committed citizens can change the world; indeed, it's the only thing that ever has.

—Margaret Mead

- Importance of a Shared Vision
- Achieving a Shared Vision
  - —Group Involvement
  - —StoryTech
- Involvement in Shared Visioning
- The Scope of Shared Visioning
- Case Studies of the Shared Visioning Process
- Summary

A shared vision is a positive force with power far beyond the image or idea it embodies. It represents an energized commitment to action aimed at creating a desired future. The commitment is tangible and real to the people who share the vision. For example, Millard Fuller was a successful businessman who, with his wife Linda, had made a fortune while in their thirties. Wondering if there was more to life, the Fullers envisioned a future in which they would dedicate their energy to eradicating homelessness and substandard housing worldwide (Fuller, 1995; Fuller & Fuller, 1990; Fuller & Scott, 1980). In 1976, the Fullers founded Habitat for Humanity. In the next twenty years, the organization expanded into a worldwide enterprise that has rehabilitated and built more than fifty thousand homes.

The process of shared visioning involves clarifying a desired future while demanding stark honesty about today's reality (Fritz, 1989). Holding these two images simultaneously produces creative tension, which then leads to action aimed at realizing the shared vision and achieving outcomes that previously seemed impossible.

The healthy population or community envisioned by providers, consumers, payers, and legislators can be shaped and powered by the creative tension caused by the gap between today's reality and the future shared vision. Creating a vision that will energize change will draw on leadership of people from all types of groups, organizations, institutions, communities, and systems. The potential for leadership becomes alive when a person is included and engaged in shared visioning, becomes invested in a larger purpose, and claims ownership for acting on the vision.

The process of mutually agreeing on values to be incorporated into the vision helps build trust among the stakeholders. Engaging community leaders and representative stakeholders in the process increases their commitment to the shared vision that emerges. Taking the shared vision to their community constituents may require risk-taking on the part of the community leaders, but it is an essential step in achieving a shared vision. The successful implementation of a shared vision demands commitment from the entire community.

Importance of a Shared Vision

The Information Age leads us into a new millennium, a new world of paradox and uncertainty. It is likely that the strategies and tools of the Postindustrial Age will not serve leaders well in the twenty-first century. The outdated image of health care organizations is that they were machines that could be understood by studying the parts and getting the parts "fixed" by executives. This static, mechanistic image must be replaced. Healthy organizations and systems in the twenty-first century will be dynamic, in a state of constant change. There will be continuous tension between stability and chaos in emerging systems. Twenty-first century leadership will recognize the necessity of vertical and horizontal integration in these evolving systems. Leaders will be responsible for promoting relationships and partnerships that spark shared visioning.

Providers alone cannot define health care adequately—the problems they see in their practices cannot be separated from the problems of the community. A new partnership of physicians, other health care providers, and community members will empower communities to examine and deal with basic behavioral, social, and environmental problems that are the root of much disease and infirmity (Manahan & Manahan, 1994).

Achieving a Shared Vision

It will take time to structure successful progress toward the shared vision. It is important to identify signposts of intermediate accomplishments and to celebrate gains.

While human and fiscal resources are necessary to achieve a shared vision, risk-taking is also essential. Millard Fuller, the founder of Habitat for Humanity, begins projects when he has 5 percent of the resources he needs (Fuller, 1995).

Collaborating partners are an important resource. Equally important is leveraging available resources by (1) letting go of nonproductive functions and services unrelated to the mission and vision, (2) creatively imagining the unimaginable, and (3) continually inviting new partners into shaping and realizing the vision. The process of achieving a shared vision can take many forms. Two successful strategies, group involvement and the StoryTech process, are described below.

Group Involvement

Trust among participants is essential. When the participants have confidence in the leadership and in the ability of fellow participants, they can proceed toward implementation of the action steps identified in the visioning process. Leaders need to allocate resources and ensure timely, effective implementation of program design in order to move the organization or system toward the vision.

It is the responsibility of leadership to provide a framework for group development of a vision. The organization's guiding principles need to be articulated. The subject matter for which the vision is to be developed needs to be identified. If any boundaries need to be established, the leadership must provide those boundaries.

The interactive planning process (see Chapter 2) was presented by Russell Ackoff of the Sloan School of Management to a group of health care providers who had received a planning grant from The Robert Wood Johnson Foundation and the Pew Charitable Trust (Ackoff, 1989b). In his presentation, Ackoff described an experience he had several years before with Bell Laboratories (Ackoff, 1989a). In this exercise, engineers and managers were told to assume that the present communication system had blown up and that they had to design a whole new system. The new system could use only technology that was currently available. They were given a time frame within which they should design the system. The new system had to be designed so that key problems historically faced by telephone users would go away. They were divided into teams, and each team was assigned a major part of the system.

Ackoff explained how the design teams first explored what they wanted to achieve, such as no wrong numbers, how they worked back to the present from that end objective, and how they then designed a system that achieved the objectives. By dealing with matters in this manner, unencumbered by the realities of today's communication systems, the teams were able to determine key objectives (a vision) and then design systems that would achieve those objectives. Twenty years later, some of the systems envisioned in that process have been designed and are a part of current communication systems.

Applying this process to the present health care environment, one set of results would emerge from the visioning process if a team of managers were asked to design a system that minimized expenses for tests and procedures. The system would look different if they were asked to maximize the likelihood of a positive patient outcome, while minimizing the health care resources needed to achieve that outcome. An even different answer would be obtained if they were asked to address how we could maximize the health of a given population while controlling resource utilization. In short, the challenge, parameters, and directions issued for the team doing the visioning are vitally important. They will be among the most significant factors, along with commitment and resource availability, in determining the outcome of the process.

As the visioning process unfolds, a broad base of involvement is essential. Involvement by multiple parties ultimately leads to more support for the vision. However, too many participants will significantly slow down the process. The ultimate decision could be compromised if the group attempts to accommodate everyone's personal position. Further, with very large numbers of participants, it may not be possible to obtain personal commitment because no one individual or group needs to own the outcome. An alternative way of broadening the base of involvement can be achieved by encouraging the active participants to discuss the process within their own stakeholder settings and then bring input to the visioning process at a subsequent meeting.

It is also important to be aware of conflicts of interest or vested interest among potential stakeholders. Parties with too much at stake personally, whose personal incentives run counter to the incentives of the overall organization, can create major difficulties in the visioning process and can compromise outcomes.

Once finalized, goals designed to move the organization toward the vision are necessary. The stakeholders involved in the visioning process, or some other group, can design the goals. The important point is not to stop with a vision; the vision needs to be converted into action plans for the vision to be realized. Goal-setting requires commitment and accountability.

StoryTech

A shared vision can also be created by using the StoryTech process.

> StoryTech is a self-guided process...a simulation modeling...as well as a powerful preplanning, visioning, and strategic tool for management. It provides a strong and renewable link between individual and organizational visions of the future, and links these directly to current activities and plans. (Harkins & Gordon, 1993, p. 1)

StoryTech uses the unique insights, wisdom, creativity, common sense, and intimate knowledge developed through life experiences or organizational roles.

StoryTech was developed by Arthur Harkins, a futurist, StoryTech consultant, and Professor of Sociology and Education. The methodology grew out of his work in using stories to understand people's perspectives as well as interviews with Japanese industrial and academic leaders about their use of imaging and long-range planning. StoryTech has been used successfully with clients, especially with clients who abused chemical substances, to help them envision a life without chemical substances and a path to that life (Harkins & Gordon, 1993).

The process uses various prompts to encourage people to share their stories, and it creates a setting in which people are asked to envision something. The facilitator usually begins by stating what year it is, where the person is located, and what the person is probably doing and wearing. Then the person is asked to answer two or three questions—in this case, about healthy communities in the future. Six to nine stories would be requested so as to provide data about the many factors that can affect the health of communities.

The second part of StoryTech refers to techniques for analyzing the data and creating a story that is representative of the many stories related to the one prompt. The StoryTech process requires money to pay a consultant/facilitator to develop the prompts for the stories and possibly to pay someone to transcribe the data and perform a preliminary analysis. Time is needed to review the data and create meaning from it.

This methodology can be used in either heterogeneous or homogeneous groups. The more the group members get to know one another and share their stories, the richer the story data becomes. The visioning process is facilitated, and a shared vision emerges.

It is critically important to include all the people from whom one needs to hear. For example, consumers of health care must be consulted. All the people who will be affected by strategies and decisions emerging from the vision need to be part of the process from the beginning.

It is essential to implement the vision immediately. As Harkins reminds participants, the future is now; it does not begin in two or three years. For some groups, change is a slow process, and it may take years to reach the agreed-upon vision. For other groups, the need to change has been recognized for some time, and with greater readiness for change, the vision can be reached more quickly. But in either case, implementation should begin immediately. Eggenberger and Huntley (1999) have described the outcomes of this process in terms of goals and guiding principles.

Involvement in Shared Visioning

As the shared visioning process evolves, more people and constituencies can become involved. Leaders should continuously articulate the vision and empower people to shape and implement it. A rural consortium funded through The Robert Wood Johnson Foundation/Pew Charitable Trusts national initiative, Strengthening Hospital Nursing: A Program to Improve Patient Care, provides an illustration of the importance of involving as many as possible in the process (Donahoe & Kohles, 1996). Also see Appendix A.

A nurse-managed regional health center, which was developed in collaboration with community-based providers, public health agencies, a state university, and professional associations, has opened new doors for services to clients. This center for the uninsured and underinsured provides a setting for learning by nurses, physicians, dentists, providers of complementary therapies, faculty, and students in nursing and the health sciences. The center has also become a catalyst for increased involvement of physicians and dentists in providing needed health care to the uninsured and underinsured. Through shared visioning by health and medical services personnel, health care consumers, and educators, a new model for providing basic health services to underserved persons has been developed. The model seeks to integrate the best of business principles, social justice, and social benefits. It enables participating partners to carry out fiscal responsibilities to the whole community, which assures the community's important role in decision making related to the health of its members.

Many other projects have evolved as administrators, faculty, physicians, directors, middle managers, nurses, and other lead workers participated in shared visioning activities. As they returned to their own department, practice, unit, service, organization, or community, they brought new tools gained from the shared visioning process. The vision was shared and further shaped according to their unique culture and environment. A ripple effect has occurred, with the vision becoming increasingly more dynamic and inclusive. Grant funds have provided seed money and consultation for interdisciplinary service and education innovation projects, which have supported local shared visioning activities. Examples of shared visioning projects include:

- Visioning for health care planning by board members and medical staff of hospitals in three communities
- Interdisciplinary education for team members providing behavioral health services for clients with dual diagnosis problems
- Organizational culture change through innovations in care delivery systems, grounded in decentralized decision making at the operational level
- Implementation of case management programs
- Improved services for and communication with victims of sexual assault
- Collaborative initiatives to address violence and its effect on children
- Development and implementation of a regional continuing health education program
- Education for regional providers to strengthen eldercare
- Provision of hospice services in a rural county
- Resource guide for regional oncology resources
- Faith-health ministry through parish nursing in congregations in nine counties
- Interdisciplinary education for crisis intervention and grief counseling

By engaging community leaders, shared visioning has been extended to include the regional planning commission, the business community, and a regional alliance of providers. Participants representing the regional commission, whose historic focus had been on agricultural, environmental, transportation and industrial issues, assumed leadership for regional rural health strategic planning through sponsorship of annual strategic planning events.

The Scope of Shared Visioning

As systems thinking demonstrates, when two or more people share personal visions, a new shared vision greater than the sum of the individual parts will emerge. To describe this phenomenon, Senge (1990) uses the metaphor of a hologram, in which interacting light sources create a three-dimensional image. In a shared visioning process, each person leaves the process with a whole image, a sense of engagement and commitment to the emerging shared vision. The person has been changed through participating in the process and now has a commitment to a larger purpose.

When leaders articulate a vision of regionwide quality, cost-effective patient and family-centered care, they create the opportunity to engage their employees and other colleagues in developing a shared vision around the kind of health care system they want to build for the future. Imagination flows, and the boundaries of the possible expand. Shared visioning promotes creativity and risk-taking while it rewards divergent and constructively critical dialogue. At the same time, it embraces playfulness and humor. Ultimately, it will provide a framework for creating the desired health care system.

On a larger scale, health care systems that involve many partners within a region, the nation, or the world need a shared vision to develop and grow. When the shared vision is founded on guiding principles and values, it unleashes the potential for developing a health care system that will achieve the goal of healthy people, healthy communities, and a healthy world community in the twenty-first century.

Case Studies of the Shared Visioning Process

Immanuel St. Joseph's–Mayo Health System is a rural regional hospital in a city of under fifty thousand inhabitants. It is geographically located an equal distance from the Twin Cities (Minneapolis and St. Paul) and Rochester, Minnesota. It is the sole hospital in the community and has a history of collaboration with smaller neighboring community hospitals.

The board of directors and members of the medical staff began their efforts to achieve a shared vision by exploring the preferred future in strategic planning sessions. Over the previous five years, Immanuel St. Joseph's–Mayo Health System had used the shared visioning process with all levels of employees, consumer focus groups, and representatives of a broad spectrum of local and regional stakeholders. Board and medical staff members had already participated with others in StoryTech.

Shared visioning led to the visualization of an integrated health care system that incorporated, at a minimum, community services, ambulatory diagnostic and treatment services, physician services, inpatient acute care, and home health care. The group assembled for the visioning task also recognized there would be continued pressure from third-party payers. Involvement in a more complete system that included tertiary care, a stronger economic base, and better negotiations with external parties would enhance the organization's ability to serve.

An analysis of the situation suggested there were at least three possibilities for such affiliations. The best of those alternatives was a locally integrated health care delivery system. Discussions with physician practice groups revealed that they intended to maintain their independence, so local integration was not feasible. Market research consultants then asked the key stakeholders—city and regional residents—where they would prefer to go for health care if they needed to leave the community. An assessment of community preferences and analysis of how the organization could maximize collaboration with local physicians led to the decision that integration with the Mayo Health System made the most sense.

The Mayo Health System and the regional hospital discussed their respective goals for an affiliation and quickly found the goals were essentially identical. A review of each other's principles showed that both organizations shared similar philosophies, leading to the conclusion an affiliation would be in the best interest of the Mayo Health System as well as the regional health care facility. After several months of discussion, the affiliation was implemented and directions for the future were set.

There was strong community support for the decision to affiliate with the Mayo Health System. That support has continued. The assumption that collaboration would be most feasible with local physician practices under a Mayo Health System umbrella has also been validated. Plans have been developed to build on local services and enhance the ability of the regional organization to serve the needs of area residents. Visioning that involved all key stakeholders identified directions that made the most sense for this community. The pursuit of that vision is serving the community well and will be instrumental in maximizing the benefits to those who now have access to national and international leadership in health care.

In another case, shared visioning has resulted in the development of a community-based project to sustain senior citizens in their homes. Using the model developed by the Living at Home–Block Nurse Program in St. Paul, Minnesota (Jamison, 1996), volunteers work with the nursing staff to provide service and expertise as needed. Volunteers provide transportation for shopping or clinic appointments, home maintenance assistance, lawn and yard care, tax preparation, banking, and other financial support. Home health nurses provide assessment and monitoring of medications and treatments, as well as coordination of total care. The shared vision has become a reality, with more than 500 people able to remain in their homes because of the services provided. A shared vision of a senior health clinic housed in a senior apartment complex emerged when faculty members, staff in the housing authority, home health nurses, and community volunteers worked together. Junior and senior nursing students consult with their faculty and one another in the care of their clients at the clinic. Blood pressure screening, foot care, ear cleaning, and skin assessment are other valued services provided. In addition, teaching about eye care, vision problems, and psychosocial care are also available. This project continues to grow, with services now being provided to four neighborhoods where the elderly population is high.

Summary

When Habitat for Humanity began, the worldwide scope of the project was only a vision. As the vision was shared with people in many diverse communities, with presidents and other world leaders, with businesses and organizations, the commitment to eradicating homelessness by providing affordable housing expanded. The vision of decent affordable housing for all that began with two people has become a compelling worldwide shared vision of people making a difference for themselves and others.

The processes of interactive planning and StoryTech will be useful in guiding communities to create a shared vision within a reality that is compatible with quality community life and the goal of healthy people and communities. As Margaret Mead taught, groups of thoughtful, organized, and committed citizens using these processes will make a difference locally, regionally, and nationally.

REFERENCES

Aadalen, S. P. (Ed.). (1996). *Health Bond: Building opportunities new directions.* Mankato, MN: Health Bond.

Ackoff, R. L. (1989a). Executive summaries—The circular organization: An update. *Academy of Management Executive, 3,* 11–16.

Ackoff, R. L. (1989b). Presentation at Strengthening Hospital Nursing: A Program to Improve Patient Care Education Program—Phase I, Education Conference for SHNP Planning Grantees, Orlando, FL.

Bartlett, J. (1992). *Familiar quotations: A collection of passages, phrases, and proverbs.* Boston: Little & Brown.

Donahoe, B. & Kohles, M. K. (1996). *Celebrating the journey: A final report.* St. Petersburg, FL: Strengthening Hospital Nursing: A Program to Improve Patient Care.

Eggenberger, S. K. and Huntley, M. I. (1999). Envisioning health care using a StoryTech process with continuing education participants. *The Journal of Continuing Education in Nursing* 30(6), 246–253.

Fritz, R. (1989). *The path of least resistance.* New York: Fawcett-Columbine.

Fuller, M. (1995). *A simple decent place to live: The building realization of Habitat for Humanity.* Dallas: Word Publishing.

Fuller, M. & Fuller, L. (1990). *The excitement is building.* Dallas: Word Publishing.

Fuller, M. & Scott, D. (1980). *Love in the mortar joints—The story of Habitat for Humanity.* Americus, GA: Associated Press, New Win Publishing, Inc.

Harkins, A. & Gordon, S. (1993). Futures in substance abuse damage control: Development for personal recovery alternatives through guided story telling. *Futurics: A Quarterly Journal of Futures Research 17,* 1–2.

Jamison, M. (1996). Grass roots efforts: Nurses involved in the political process. In E. L. Cohen (Ed.). *Nurse case management in the twenty-first century,* pp. 12–17. St. Louis, MO: Mosby.

Manahan, W. & Manahan, D. (1994). The nurse as the primary health care practitioner. *Holistic Medicine, 4,* 2–3.

Senge, P. M. (1990). *The fifth discipline: The art and practice of the learning organization.* New York: Doubleday Currency.

CHAPTER

5 Culture Change

ALICE WEYDT

LYNETTE FROEHLICH

SHIRLEY RAETZ

Some men see things as they are and say "why?"
I dream things that never were and say "why not?"

—George Bernard Shaw

- From Primary Care to Community Primary Health Care
- Leadership for Culture Change
- A Case Study of Culture Change
- Outcomes of Culture Change
- Summary

Organizational culture change is essential for building individual, community, and regional health. Throughout the twentieth century, the illness care delivery system has made incredible advances. Organ transplants, genetic engineering, antibiotics, and other pharmaceutical discoveries are but a few examples of the victories achieved in the ongoing struggle against illness and death.

Historically, consumers of health care services took a passive role in managing their health care and placed blind trust in the health care system. Health care remained a mystery, and the issues of health were left for the professionals to decide. Health care professionals took great pride in their clinical competence. Their time and energy were devoted to learning the technology and illness care processes of diagnosis and treatment. Individual disciplines tended to isolate themselves and did not value each other's contributions to the well-being of the patient. Turf issues and empire building ran rampant as organizations departmentalized around functions. Health care bureaucracies flourished, and the patient and family became lost in the maze of conflicting systems.

Health care administration, especially in hospitals, traditionally has had a hierarchical structure with top-down leadership. Hospital administrators made decisions about operations that affected the providers of services, as well as the patients and families, with little understanding of how the decisions affected clinical outcomes. Struggles between clinical focus and financial incentives created an environment of mistrust and barriers to valuing one another's expertise. Consequently, health care systems have become reimbursement driven rather than clinically driven.

Society has given the health care industry a clear message that the cost of services cannot continue to escalate. Cost-containing efforts have resulted in capitation and managed care systems. There is frustration within health care as resources shrink and the demands for health care services increase. Consumers, on the other hand, become frustrated when they pay high prices but do not receive the service or results that they expect. Legislators and third-party payers look for compromise in resource allocation rather than revamping the entire health care system. To truly address health care concerns, everyone must change.

Becoming a proactive society that takes responsibility for health outcomes requires a major paradigm shift by health care providers and consumers. To merely modify the existing system only perpetuates a convoluted form of illness care. Basic philosophical changes are needed to change the entire system. As with any system, however, there is a desire for homeostasis in health care. In an attempt to control and predict, health care providers have missed the opportunity to create a holistic health care system and have created a system focused on disease or discomfort. Efforts to change the health care system are likely to encounter resistance from those who are making the most profit from the current system.

In the last half of the twentieth century, America became an increasingly mobile society. There are few large extended families living within defined geographical boundaries. Connectedness, or being part of a family system, has become difficult. Families of today are diverse, and many individuals have no family ties. When there is no family to provide health care, additional pressure is placed on health care providers to find someone to provide the care needed.

People seek health care in a variety of settings from a diverse group of health care providers who may or may not share information. This sets the stage for enormous duplication and fragmentation of services. One strategy to address the gaps in the system is through regionalization of health care, which will allow specialty care to be provided to a larger portion of the population. Regional health care networks offer the promise of reducing duplication of effort and fragmentation of care through enhanced communication and collaboration. The focus changes from solo practitioners and singular relationships between a physician and patient to an integrated system that better addresses the health care needs of people and communities.

The consumer will force culture change on the twenty-first century health care delivery system. Many consumers are medically savvy, have electronic access to information, and search for answers independently. They will demand more involvement in their care. However, individual consumers may have less control than their health insurance company, and price and quality, rather than loyalty to a particular practitioner, may determine who is selected for health care services. In some markets, consumers have strongly objected to being forced to change providers, and consumer choice has prevailed.

Today's health care leaders must be aware of the values and ethics of this new generation of consumers and must become involved within their communities. Health care leaders must not only assess current needs of communities, they also need to try to articulate the future. Leaders must be visionaries in order to build healthy communities.

Flexibility to change seems like a small thing. Most leaders would say they already possess this quality. But many within the community disagree and see themselves as victims of inflexible leaders. Health care leaders must be able to see the opportunities, looking beyond today, and see how new technologies, new lifestyles, and new health practices will affect health care delivery. This may require leaders to change strategies and goals and be open to new possibilities, mutual trust, and respect. All members of a health care team will need to feel that this trust and respect are genuine. Team members at any level will not commit to working together or taking responsibility if there is any doubt. Leaders must be seen as members of the team, concerned for all other team members.

From Primary Care to Community Primary Health Care

The community primary health care model is part of a paradigm that can create a new vision of initiatives to foster healthy people and communities. A transformation at all levels is necessary to change from an illness care model to a community primary health care model (see Chapter 2). Individuals will need to take responsibility for their health throughout life. Families and communities will need to work together to provide support for healthy lifestyles. Health care professionals will need to understand their new roles in promoting health. Leaders of health care providers and payers will need to accept this new focus and incorporate incentives into their organizations and health systems.

Authority and responsibility will need to be transferred to patients and their families, empowering them to make informed decisions about their own health and lifestyle. Relationships among patients and their families, providers, administrators, and payers will change as this shift occurs. New systems must be created so that all can become active partners in designing and building on clinical competencies for ideal community primary health care.

Education for professionals in the community primary health care model must address (1) the philosophy of health along a continuum from birth to death, including health promotion, disease prevention, and individual responsibilities for health; (2) the importance of being good stewards of resources; (3) interdisciplinary collaboration that values the expertise of all members of the health care team; and (4) ethical considerations in an environment of limited resources.

The ultimate goal of the community primary health care model is for people to become empowered to accept responsibility for their own health. Technological breakthroughs provide us with the tools to monitor health status over the lifespan. At the basic level, software programs track medications, procedures, and lifestyle choices. At a more sophisticated level, these programs can provide warnings of adverse interactions or prior negative reactions as new medications are proposed. The individual could then be advised of preventive testing or lifestyle changes that might be beneficial. Individuals would have access to their own health records and learn how their choices affect their health. In every interaction with the health care system, the individual would be given more information about and support for a healthful lifestyle.

The building blocks for healthy communities are healthy individuals and healthy families at all economic levels of society. Although an emphasis on individual responsibility is important, society must also provide population-based public health services for the health of its citizens. As noted by Shoultz and Hatcher,

> a multi-sectorial approach that requires partnership, collaboration, and community involvement and fosters development of self-reliance—if all of these critical precursors of health are ignored and only personal health services are delivered—then the opportunities to develop healthier communities in which policies and action in other sectors work in tandem with health services to promote health and prevent disease will be lost. Ethical professional behavior demands a primary health care approach that includes and goes beyond personal health services. (1997, p. 24)

Leadership for Culture Change

A commitment to a shared decision-making partnership involving consumers and providers of health care will be the desired culture for the twenty-first century. In such a culture, leaders will need to model desired behaviors and set clear expectations about achieving the vision and mission of a community primary health care model.

Cultures will not change if leadership doesn't internalize and accept the desired changes. Leaders will need to use role modeling, engage in collaborative behaviors, and set clear expectations about achieving the vision and mission. Leaders will have to "walk the talk" and accept responsibility for the organization's culture change.

Leaders often feel threatened by changes in culture because power has to be shared; power and control can no longer reside in a few. Leaders will become students as they go beyond their organizations to facilitate change. Leaders and staff will be confident enough to risk making mistakes as new leadership skills are acquired. Education and training resources are essential for this transformation to occur.

Culture change will demand new learning for people at all levels. The sense of responsibility and accountability for health will need to be fostered and nurtured throughout people's lives. Only when this new community primary health care model has been incorporated into the culture of the people, the providers, and the leaders, will there be lifestyle changes.

The first phase will come when leaders recognize that they have to change themselves first. Admitting shortcomings and incorporating new behaviors into daily practice will feel risky. These feelings are not unique to leadership, because the change will affect staff, patients, and families as well. As emphasis shifts from financial outcomes to clinical outcomes, the knowledge base will also shift. Consumer involvement in decision making that is based on knowledge of clinical outcomes data will require changes in the way care is delivered.

Health care will no longer be viewed as a series of tasks but rather as a process that requires integration and collaboration of systems within an organization as well as across the life continuum. Involving staff members as partners in creating the desired future will help them buy into the shift from task to process. No change is sustained without horizontal pressure. Staff members have a larger influence on one another than leaders have on staff. It is vital, then, for staff members to become involved in creating the desired future. Change at the grassroots level empowers staff to take on leadership roles and start leading their leaders.

There are three tiers of leadership development that will affect culture change. First, leaders, direct care providers, and patients and their families will have responsibility in creating new systems that will meet future challenges. Each individual will become an active partner in determining an ideal community primary health care model.

Second, staff providing the care will need information about finances and will need to become stewards of resources. In addition to an emphasis on care processes and use of technology, staff will be involved in shared visioning and strategic planning and must know how to use the interactive planning process (Ackoff, 1986; 1989).

Third, consumers will need to take an active role in managing their own health care. People can no longer assume that health care services are a right and that health care providers will make decisions for them and their families.

A transformation at all three levels is necessary to transition from an illness/disease model to a community primary health care model. Administrative leaders will need to share financial expertise in order to maximize health care resources. New strategies and a shared vision will need to be developed as health care goes beyond the walls of traditional health care organizations and becomes integrated within the community and region.

The importance of physician leadership cannot be overstated. Physicians will need to be committed to a philosophy of community primary health care. Physicians with administrative experience can bridge the clinical/financial perspective. Both interests are served when ensuring positive outcomes and fiscal viability. Understanding the financial implications in clinical practice allows the most effective research-based care at the lowest cost. Currently, conflicting financial incentives between physicians, hospitals, and third-party payers interfere with this goal.

Strategies that leaders can use to influence culture change include interactive planning (see Chapter 2), regionalization (see Chapter 3), and shared visioning (see Chapter 4). A case study of culture change illustrates these strategies.

A Case Study of Culture Change

Immanuel St. Joseph's Hospital (ISJ) in Mankato, Minnesota, was a traditional hierarchical hospital. In the 1980s, it began to explore new ways to collaborate and form partnerships with medical practices and other rural hospitals in south-central Minnesota. The efforts resulted in a lawsuit by the state attorney general for conflict of interest, fraud, and restraint of trade. Although the lawsuit was settled out of court, hospital and physician representatives had become hesitant about further joint ventures.

In 1989, the Health Bond project (see Appendix A) created a framework to explore opportunities for collaboration and forming of partnerships. New skills were developed, and roles shifted. Health Bond facilitated collaboration and provided opportunities to learn about and value an interdisciplinary team. This work started at the grassroots level, where patients, families, and staff started to ask questions about how the system could improve. The team went beyond the walls of the hospital to community organizations and agencies.

In 1995, Mankato experienced a meningitis outbreak. When the third case was diagnosed, the state epidemiologist met with the school district, local and state government officials, health care providers, and community relations experts to discuss how to address this serious situation. The stakeholders were brought together for a common vision of protecting and educating a vulnerable and frightened community. It took only a few hours for a plan of action to be implemented.

Initially, the outbreak seemed to be restricted to one of the three high schools, and an immunization program was confined to those students. As additional cases appeared and a death resulted from the meningitis bacteria, the immunization program was expanded. All Mankato area residents aged two through twenty-nine were encouraged to be immunized with meningococcal vaccine and to receive an antibiotic. Immanuel–St. Joseph's Hospital, the Mankato public schools, Blue Earth County Human Services, the Nicollet County health department, the regional epidemiologist, county and city elected officials, state legislators, physicians from two local clinics, nursing faculty and students from the local university and technical college, together with numerous community public, private, and voluntary organizations, all collaborated and cooperated with the Minnesota Department of Health to provide a mass immunization program for the population at risk. Hospital staff initiated the process but stepped back to let collaboration among the stakeholders occur. Collaboration turned a potentially dangerous situation into an opportunity for community growth and development.

What happened during this crisis should happen on a routine basis. Traditional ways of addressing concerns were set aside. People listened and valued one another's expertise. All participants remarked that this kind of spirit should exist on a day-to-day basis. They also agreed with the opinion expressed in the *Los Angeles Times* (see Appendix C) that the aggressive response was the correct one.

This was a powerful experience for those who lived it. What was learned is that collaboration removes barriers that were previously thought impossible to address. Michael T. Osterholm, the state epidemiologist, described the experience this way:

> The public health crisis was addressed through the collective efforts of the local community, area public health agencies, the school district, post-secondary institutions, elected officials, and community leaders. These efforts represented the very best in community leadership. As we have said throughout, your community was negotiating uncharted waters during this outbreak. The manner in which the entire community has responded will serve as a gold standard for the next community that faces such an outbreak. Many of you will be called upon to provide advice in the future, and to help guide the public health response to similar crises across the country. ("Meningitis Outbreak," 1995)

Outcomes of Culture Change

An empowered culture accepts responsibility for outcomes. Freedom is a byproduct of this process. Although many in American society have a nostalgic view of the family doctor who cared for a person from cradle to grave, who knew that person's entire family and community, and who had enough life experience to provide wisdom and comfort when medicine fell short, few people have firsthand experience of such a relationship. This view, however, holds a valuable image that needs to be translated into a contemporary framework.

For many reasons, consumers rarely have had a chance to see the same health care providers over time. The explosion of knowledge makes it impossible for providers to have current knowledge of all aspects of health care. Providers and consumers rarely remain in one community throughout their lives. Changing insurance plans may force a transfer to a new provider even if people don't leave their community. As health care enters a new century, the benefits of the old-time family doctor's continuity need to be carried forward in technology and policy.

Technological breakthroughs are becoming commonplace and mundane. The challenge is to harness the capabilities of technology while preserving the human perspective. Computers can support data continuity. Providers miles apart can be linked in seconds, and masses of data can be transmitted quickly and accurately in the form of words, pictures, and sound. Consumers can also keep their own database, with software programs that record health information from birth throughout life. The challenges facing this technological continuity are privacy, data overload, and compatibility between different hardware and software systems. Health care has been moving outside the hospital walls for the past decade. Now data will be moving outside as well, to an integrated electronic health record that will be accessed whenever or wherever a person enters the health care system.

Policy decisions will require sound input from a health care community and stakeholders who are willing to grapple with the larger issues. Fragmented solutions to individual problems serve only to snarl the web of health care. Petty turf wars will serve neither consumers nor providers. Providers, hospitals, health plans, and allied health services need to bring expertise as well as a willingness to understand the needs of other players so as to assist clients to make the necessary transitions within an integrated health care delivery system. No individual will be able to arbitrarily control the situation. Systems will be negotiated on multiple levels, and it will be critical to keep the needs and desires of individuals and communities as the primary focus. As systems improve, consumer expectations will rise and stimulate competition to further improve the process of health care delivery.

Systems will need to offer a variety of choices to those they serve. Without choice, options diminish. If the options are not diverse or readily available, they will not be utilized, and the potential to reach a higher level of wellness may not be realized.

There will also be an increasing proportion of care directed toward chronic health problems. In the twentieth century, acute problems have demanded rapid diagnosis and treatment, with relatively little follow-up care. When an individual was sick, treatment either resolved the issue without long-term consequences or, if there were sequelae, they were left to the individual and the family to manage. Unless all antibiotic resources are lost to resistant strains, or other unforeseen demands for acute care develop, the proportion of care directed at chronic conditions will continue to rise. This is obvious when one considers the effect of aging in our society. The emphasis will move from an illness/disease orientation to how to move people back to health and well-being. Prevention of chronic disabling conditions that are unresponsive to acute interventions will become critical.

Summary

The focus of medicine in the twentieth century has been on care of acute illnesses, disease, and injuries. Now the time has come to focus on prevention, rehabilitation, and chronic illness care. What is immediately apparent is that care will not be provided by one person or even one team. There needs to be continuity as consumers move and resources are allocated to provide the best care for the regional dollar. Continuity is necessary as consumers age and find that their health care needs are different from when they were younger. The shared vision for health care in the twenty-first century will broaden with a closer look at the complexity of continuity in a community primary health care model. Interactive planning will be a helpful process in creating the new paradigm and new ways of collaborating.

REFERENCES

Ackoff, R. L. (1989). Presentation at Strengthening Hospital Nursing: A Program to Improve Patient Care Education Program—Phase I, Education Conference for SHNP Planning Grantees. Orlando, FL.

Ackoff, R. L. (1986). *Management in small doses.* New York: John Wiley and Sons.

Bartlett, J. (1992). *Familiar quotations: A collection of passages, phrases, and proverbs.* Boston: Little & Brown.

Meningitis outbreak (1995, March 16). Mankato, MN: *The Mankato Free Press* (p. 4).

Schoultz, J. and Hatcher, P. (1997). Looking beyond primary care to primary health care: An approach to community based action. *Nursing Outlook, 45,* 23–26.

CHAPTER

6 Continuum of Care

LAURIE DAHL
ALICE WEYDT
LYNETTE FROEHLICH

No one is managing the patient's transition through the system.
—Thomas W. Langfitt, M.D.
President, Pew Charitable Trusts

- The Continuum of Care Imperative
  —Interregional Care Continuum
  —Health Care Delivery System Model
  —Consumer-Focused Care
- Process to Implement Care Across the Continuum
- Strategies to Achieve a Care Continuum
  —Community Care Management
  —Nurse Case Management
  —Benefits of Nurse Case Management
  —Integrated Information Infrastructure
- Summary

The challenge for health care delivery in the twenty-first century is to develop an integrated system that serves people throughout their lives. Health care systems are currently not held accountable for consumer-centered delivery of care throughout the lifespan. Delivery systems have not recognized the multidimensional, interdependent, interpersonal, and ongoing nature of disease and disability (Bringewatt, 1995). If the human condition were static, there would be no need to define the continuum of care. Because of the dynamic changes that occur in the natural aging process and the effect of chronic illness and disabilities on health status, the continuum of care takes on paramount significance. It is in our best interest to manage disability and chronic disease through prevention and rehabilitation rather than an acute care/illness-driven approach.

The word *continuum* is a derivative of *continuous* and is defined as "an uninterrupted extension in space, time, or sequence" (*Webster's Dictionary,* 1997, p. 284). *Continuum of care* implies interdependent relationships across time, provider, and setting. Integration does not itself guarantee a continuum of care. Providers can be integrated at an operational level but still not provide a seamless system.

Literature searches reveal few endeavors that have successfully achieved integration and collaboration across the continuum of care. Although there is much discussion and activity pertaining to system networks and provider relationships, true person-centered systems focusing on health throughout the lifespan are rare. A shared vision based on common values and trust will be needed in order to shift our thinking to a community primary health care model (see Chapter 4).

Today, most strategies to improve health focus on health promotion and disease prevention. The Health Futures Institute (1993) asserts that when people live in a safe, clean environment in which they can obtain education, find employment, and generate enough income to afford housing and other basic needs, they are then empowered to take responsibility for their health. Therefore, health care providers should be involved in creating conditions for individuals and communities to feel empowered and accept responsibility for their future health.

The Continuum of Care Imperative

The need for a continuum of care has not always been acknowledged. Emphasis has been placed on containing costs, prompting the development of provider networks. The underpinnings for this endeavor have been financial motivation rather than concern for quality health outcomes. Reengineering our delivery system to minimize the effects of disease and disability is an important strategy in the development of an integrated continuum of care.

Initial efforts to improve the continuum of care within an environment of an episodic illness care system demonstrate the value of a patient-centered approach. For example, small community hospitals may send their patients to large tertiary hospitals for cardiology procedures. The length of stay at the tertiary hospital for these interventions is between one and five days, during which the patient is in pain, sedated, or preoccupied with tests and procedures. When patients return home, they need follow-up care, but they may be very far away from the tertiary hospital where they received treatment. Referral back to the community for follow-up care may have been initiated but may not reach the appropriate resources in a timely manner.

Interregional Care Continuum

A clinical pathway for heart health care has been developed and implemented across tertiary and community care to improve follow-up care (Doran, Sampson, Staus, Ahern & Schiro, 1997). The pathway has four phases:

1. The acute phase, in which a tertiary nurse care manager initiates the pathway and provides an assessment of the patient and a discharge summary to the community nurse care manager (CNCM)
2. The recovery phase, which begins the day after discharge with a visit from the CNCM and ends when the patient begins a cardiac rehabilitation program
3. The rehabilitation phase, which includes medical evaluations, a prescribed exercise program, education on modifying cardiac risk factors, and behavioral counseling by the CNCM
4. The enhancement/maintenance phase, which begins with the completion of cardiac rehabilitation and ends with the anniversary of the acute event, or when the patient has incorporated lifestyle changes into patterns of daily living.

Doran et al. (1997) based the development of this clinical pathway on Gordon's functional health patterns (1987) and the Omaha System (Martin & Scheet, 1992). The clinical pathway provides baseline scores that are used to guide practice and communication between the tertiary and community nurse case managers. Through this system of formal follow-up care and reinforcement both within and beyond the tertiary care center, patients who have had major cardiac interventions are able to experience healthier lives.

The system for communication, care delivery, managing transition, and meeting patient needs resides within individuals whose presence guarantees that needs will be met. The lesson learned is that the technology must support interregional care across the continuum.

Health Care Delivery System Model

Communication among health care delivery systems has improved with the use of computer and telecommunication technologies by hospitals, clinics, and physicians' offices. The situation will become ideal when patients and their families can be the source of their own health histories, using technology to store, transfer, and analyze health information. It is believed that patients and their families will carry health information on a computer chip that is updated each time services are provided or status changes. The information could even be translated into other languages when people move to or visit other countries.

When perspectives about the continuum of care are broadened, an integrated systems approach to health care delivery becomes essential. Even more important than the full use of technology is the acknowledgment of interdependence by separate health care delivery systems.

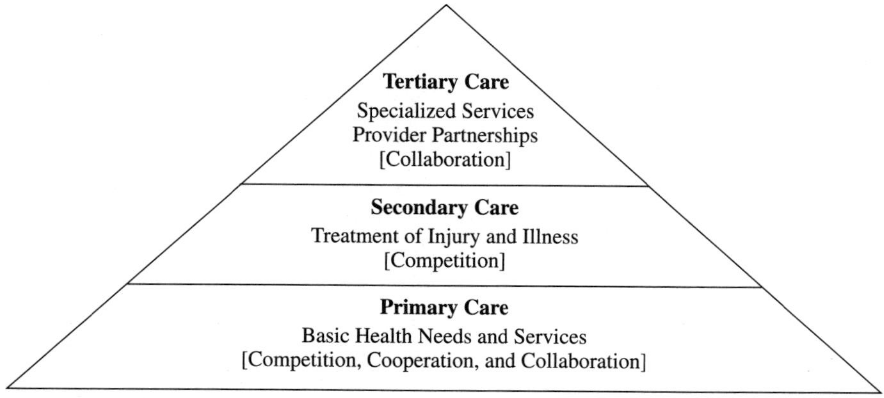

FIGURE 6.1 Health Care Delivery System Model for a Continuum of Care

Material taken from work completed through Immanuel St. Joseph's–Mayo Health System, Mankato, Minnesota, Departments of Community Health Services and Patient Care Services (1998). By permission.

Figure 6.1 illustrates the level of cooperation, collaboration, and competition among health care delivery systems as they are involved in providing primary, secondary, and tertiary care. The base of the triangle depicts primary care services used by over 85 percent of the population. Although there is competition for clients at this level, cooperation and collaboration among health care providers is necessary in order for primary care services to be available to all. Combined efforts to provide adequate prenatal care, nutrition programs, immunization clinics, and other health promotion programs to all people in a community is the foundation of a continuum of care approach.

The need for secondary and tertiary care would be eliminated in a perfect world. In the real world of health care, however, people have injuries and illnesses that must be treated. In larger communities, the consumer will have a choice of health care providers and hospitals. The middle layer of the triangle in Figure 6.1 represents the secondary care given to those who have acute and chronic illnesses. Although some communities have only one hospital, people still choose among neighboring community hospitals or alternative health care providers when they need treatment for an illness. Competition for secondary care is likely to increase in the twenty-first century, unless third-party payers gain monopolies that limit choices.

Collaboration among health care providers is necessary in order to have tertiary care available. This is represented in the top tier of Figure 6.1. Expensive diagnostic and treatment procedures cannot be available everywhere. Even though the goal is to avoid expensive specialty care, there will be demand for transplants, coronary artery bypass graft surgery, and other specialized procedures as long as resources remain available. Communities must collaborate within a region to make these services a part of the continuum of care, reducing waste and duplication of services.

A continuum of care is inherent in most managed care health plans. Managed care plans began with event-driven cost avoidance strategies. The focus is on reducing in-patient hospital days to control costs. Evolving from that have been activities addressing value improvement, with peer review and physician networks targeting resource intensity. "As managed care firms succeed in stripping out layers of cost from hospitalization reductions, delivery system consolidation, and clinical process improvement, they will have to find new strategies for creating value" (Goldsmith, Goran & Nackel, 1995). Ultimately, plans will include incentives that empower individuals, families, and communities to take responsibility for their own health, thus bringing about improvements in health within communities. Managing health risks requires vertical integration of health care systems and horizontal integration of multiple stakeholders to develop the continuum of care.

Consumer-Focused Care

Jeffrey Bauer, a health economist, espouses the need for a consumer revolution in health care in order to provide the continuum of care we have been describing. Bauer (1998) posits the following vision of the future:

- "Independent nonphysician providers will deliver a significant portion of our nation's primary care" (p. 216)
- "Pharmacies and diagnostic centers will offer consumers new opportunities for self-diagnosis and self-treatment" (p. 217)
- "The market for primary care services will develop to resemble the market for other consumer goods and services" (p. 218)
- "Physicians will assume the roles of both specialty-care providers, managers, and entrepreneurs within the new system" (p. 219)
- "Basic public health services will be delivered in many new settings" (p. 219)
- "Voluntary (tax-exempt, not-for-profit) hospitals will assume new and different roles as the institutional center of the future health care system." (p. 220)

Bauer concludes that, ultimately, Americans want healthier people from our health care system. To satisfy this desire, all health care providers must collaborate across the care continuum.

To develop an integrated continuum of care, current systems will need to be re-engineered not only structurally but also at the higher level of vision and goals. If our aim is to minimize the effects of disease and disability, then the emphasis will move away from diagnosis and treatment toward developing health and well-being. Technological advances in diagnosis and treatment will never outweigh the value of prevention of chronic disabling conditions. For instance, lung transplant technology will continue to improve, but it will never be as effective as preventing lung diseases.

Often solutions for problems in continuity are created from the perspective of the provider organizations. A referral process is set up for one provider to transfer care to another provider. The smoothest systems develop when the planners walk throughout the process from the viewpoint of the consumer or staff who are directly involved with the process. Consumer involvement will result in raised expectations, thus driving the system to continuously improve the process.

Initially, people cooperate without a clearly defined mission, structure, or planning effort. They share information but retain authority and risk little. This level of relationship is very vulnerable because outcomes are dependent on specific individuals. As more formal relationships evolve, understanding and coordination occur, resulting in longer term interactions. Authority still rests within individual organizations, so power can be an issue. The continuum of care requires true collaboration, characterized by a durable and pervasive relationship bringing separate entities together with full commitment to a common vision and values. Authority is redefined and partners share risks and outcomes (Winer, 1995). The guiding principles of customer focus, teamwork, and constant innovation become the new paradigm. Health care providers will need to start collaborating not only with each other but also with consumers and communities, to develop processes that achieve a true continuum of care.

Process to Implement Care Across the Continuum

Five phases describe the process to implement care across the continuum. These five phases are patterned after problem-solving processes within a systems context.

In the first phase, data are gathered from stakeholders. The stakeholders include the consumers of the service as well as the providers and payers. Focus groups encourage consumers and their families to tell their stories. Direct feedback from consumers provides insight into the process of care. Providers and payers often lack the consumer perspective. It is difficult to change a paradigm from within.

Once data are gathered, the second phase requires consumers, payers, and providers to assess current systems and analyze the findings in the context of the expectations of the consumer. This gap analysis, and the resulting creative tension, become the map and the motivation toward systems improvement. Creative tension is the catalyst for creating a shared vision of the desired future (Senge, 1990).

The third phase involves the identification of strategic priorities and resources required to meet identified objectives. The paradigm must shift from managing an individual's episodic illness to population-based care management with an emphasis on health. Priorities will be dictated by population needs and will vary over time and setting.

Implementation teams are brought together in the fourth phase. These are transdisciplinary teams that span organizations, communities, and health care systems to meet the needs identified in the strategic priorities. Adequate resources will need to be allocated to implement major systems improvements. Traditional thinking must not become a barrier to creative innovations.

Essential to the implementation process is the evaluation of the effectiveness and efficiency of care across the continuum. In the final phase, it is important to revisit the original vision in order to evaluate the outcomes of the change. Has the desired outcome been achieved? Measuring outcomes is unfamiliar to us. The question that begs to be answered is whether the health of those being served has been improved, and on what basis the determination is made. The effect of the changes on care across the continuum can be measured only by an integrated information system. Likewise, the degree to which an integrated delivery system affects the overall health of the community is dependent on an infrastructure that allows the electronic transfer of individual and population-based health information.

Strategies to Achieve a Care Continuum

To develop a continuum of care, more is needed than good intentions and adequate use of technology. The people who are designing and using the systems must be involved in what Hargrove (1998) has labeled "creative collaboration." Hargrove outlines the "recipe for creative collaboration" as follows:

- "Step 1. Make a declaration of impossibility (something you want to accomplish)" (p. 34)
- "Step 2. Bring extraordinary combinations of people together who can make the impossible a reality" (p. 34)
- "Step 3. Build a shared understood goal that transforms the possibility into a live project" (p. 35)
- "Step 4. Do a 'what's so' (complete factual analysis) about what you want to achieve" (p. 36)
- "Step 5. Identify what's missing that, if provided, could produce a breakthrough." (p. 37)

The three examples outlined in the following sections use varying strategies to follow the above steps. These three examples illustrate the need for collaboration to achieve a true continuum of care.

Community Care Management

Community care management requires partnerships between health care providers, individual consumers, families, and neighborhoods. One example of a model that integrates community care management is Teams Across the Continuum for Systems Improvement (TACSI). In Figure 6.2, the care continuum is represented in the oblong circle above the three triangles. These three triangles are aspects of one interdependent system that supports the continuum. They are interconnected by the nurse case manager, who helps the client and family negotiate services that meet their health care

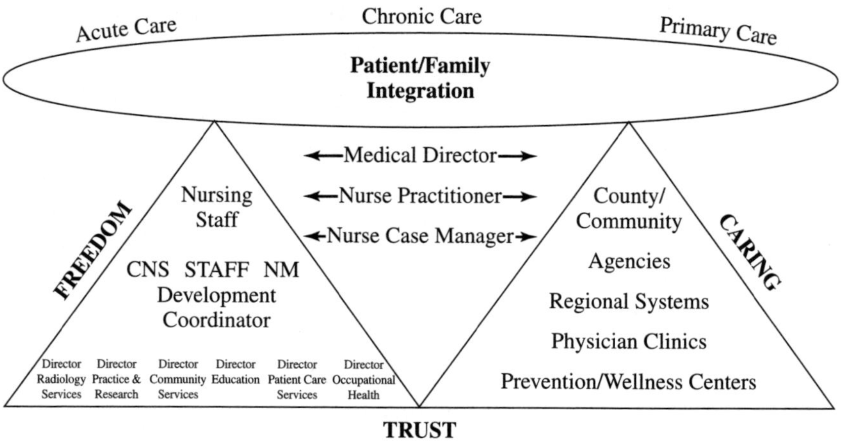

FIGURE 6.2 TACSI: Teams Across the Continuum for Systems Improvement

Material taken from work completed through Immanuel St. Joseph's–Mayo Health System, Mankato, Minnesota, Departments of Community Services and Patient Care Services (1999). By permission.

needs (Cohen, 1996). Nurse practitioners provide direct health care services as well as screening, education, and referral to the medical director when appropriate. Acute care occurs within the walls of hospitals and is supported by an interdisciplinary team with specialized skills in meeting acute care needs. Helping clients and families navigate a complex environment is part of the team's responsibility.

Primary care occurs outside the acute care setting and focuses on prevention and wellness. Community and regional resources are tapped to minimize the effects of a potential chronic disease. The goal would be to reduce the utilization of acute services.

The three triangles are components of one integrated system. Freedom, trust, and caring are the foundation for clients and families to develop and initiate health care strategies that meet their needs. Freedom, trust, and caring are also the foundations for organizations to develop an integrated system. These three concepts are described by McBeth and Weydt as the "essence of an innovative collaborative delivery system" (1996, p. 105). Freedom to explore options available to each consumer, patient, and family is the essence of the first concept. Trust cannot occur unless there is freedom to learn about the potential. Caring is the vehicle that communicates to clients and their families that they are valued and understood.

Nurse Case Management

Nurse case management is a strategy that is evolving nationally to coordinate care as individual and family members transition through organizations and systems. Its use has improved clinical outcomes, reduced fragmentation and duplication, and reduced system costs (Cohen, 1996). Nurse case management addresses the continuum of care, emphasizing an individual's—and the person's support system's—responsibility for the person's health. Understanding the values of clients and their support system is vital to mutually setting goals. Building a trusting relationship between the nurse case manager and the client fosters client independence, creating options for informed choices. Studies across the country demonstrate that, using nurse case management, client satisfaction increases, complex conditions stabilize, earlier interventions reduce the number of acute hospital admissions and the duration of hospitalization, and quality of life improves (Cohen, 1996). Three independent studies from 1995 through 1998 at Immanuel St. Joseph's–Mayo Health System demonstrated a savings of over a million dollars in system costs following the integration of nurse case management into the continuum of care. Three diverse case scenarios demonstrate these outcomes. These three cases are composites, and the names used do not represent actual clients. These three cases from Immanuel St. Joseph's–Mayo Health System provide examples of the variety of services used across the continuum of care.

Complex Chronic Illness Case Scenario. Chester was eighty-eight years old and had been diagnosed as having spastic bladder, hypertension, and congestive heart failure. He was a frequent visitor to the emergency room (ER) and made multiple calls to his primary physician. He frequently saw different physicians when he came into the clinic or ER.

The nurse case manager (NCM) received two telephone referrals—one from the primary physician, the other from an emergency room nurse and the ER medical director. Medication, diet education, and systems assessments were completed by the NCM. Chester did not meet Medicare requirements for home care services, but the hospital's commitment to a continuum of care for its clients, through the NCM, meant that appropriate care was available for Chester.

The first NCM visit took place in the emergency room, since that was where Chester was on that day. The NCM introduced herself and explained her role as a nurse who could partner with him to help him obtain more direct care from his primary physician and make fewer trips to the emergency room. Chester's response was, "I don't suppose you can get me home, they won't let me go unless I can find a ride home, my wife doesn't drive." The NCM responded by saying she could give Chester a ride home and that they would visit on the way. Chester replied, "Huh, you can come in and meet Marjorie, since you're going to be my nurse."

Initially, the NCM visited once a week, monitoring Chester's vital signs and weight, performing a partial cardiac and respiratory assessment, providing education regarding his diet, medication, and disease process. As a team, the primary physician, Chester, and NCM were able to develop a plan and set parameters for his medication regimen. Through education by the NCM, Chester learned about his body and the purposes of his treatment plan. Previously Chester was labeled a nuisance because he made so many calls to the physician and then did not follow instructions. Now when Chester calls, he has his data ready for the NCM.

Chester's utilization of the ER has decreased by 90 percent, and telephone calls to the physician have decreased by 75 percent. Chester's wife, Marjorie, also had numerous health issues. By having a NCM working with her, the primary physician has been kept abreast of changes and concerns in a timely manner for both Chester and Marjorie. Hospitalizations have been appropriate. Home care services were initiated when needed. Volunteers have been enlisted to help with household chores and nutritional needs. The common thread throughout this change has been the consistent connection among Chester, Marjorie, one primary physician, and one NCM.

Chemical Dependency Case Scenario. The chemical dependency unit at a midwestern hospital has a unique program to address the needs of chemically dependent women who are either pregnant or have young children. The Renaissance Program provides resources and support to encourage personal growth and a new beginning by removing barriers to treatment and promoting recovery. The goal is to empower women to maximize their individual wellness. The NCM plays a vital role in their treatment process. The following is one woman's story.

Ann was a twenty-four-year-old pregnant woman with two children at home, one of whom had a disability. Ann's husband did not provide financial support and was abusive, so Ann had obtained a restraining order against him. She was very angry during her first two weeks in the program. She kept saying, "All I need help with is my children and transportation." She expressed frustration about trying to take care of her children with no outside help. Child protection services became involved because of physical altercations with her spouse and situations involving alcohol.

While in treatment, she gave birth, and then brought her newborn to aftercare groups. Other women were very accepting of her, her children, and her situation. Her aftercare focused on parenting classes and provided transportation funds so that she could get to appointments, classes, and the grocery store. The NCM connected Ann to support services in the community.

Ann has now been moved to inactive status, receiving infrequent follow-up calls. She participates in a parenting program and receives assistance for her disabled son. She receives housing assistance so she and her children can live in a three-bedroom duplex. Ann relates:

> People tell me I look and act differently; they talk to me now. They think it's because I had a baby, but I know it's because my self-esteem is better. I feel like a part of society, not just one of those welfare mothers. I can go to the park with all my children, visit with other parents, my children have room to play. My children walk with their shoulders straighter. Even my Dad sees the difference and he sits and talks with me for a while. I know I'm better, stronger. And if I get in trouble with drinking, I know I can call up and get help. I know where I can get help now if I need it.

Ann had been so full of anger that she pushed people away. As she learned new communication skills and had some small successes, the anger was transformed into assertiveness. She has become empowered to make changes that have improved her health.

Maternal-Child Case Scenario. An NCM was referred to see a family whose female twins were born prematurely at thirty-four weeks. After a long hospital stay, complicated by what was believed to be an infection acquired there, the infants were finally discharged to home, with six medications and an apnea monitor. Home care nurses followed the family for the first few weeks to monitor vital signs, weight, medication compliance, apnea spells, feeding, and the parents' ability to cope with twins as well as their other three children. After a few weeks, the insurance company denied any further home visits, stating that the parents could take the babies to the physician's office as needed. There was no understanding or concern about the home situation. At that time, the NCM told the parents about the external nurse case management program. The parents were receptive, and the twins were admitted to the program.

The twins are now one year old. The NCM saw the family through an allergic reaction to a DPT shot, visits to the physician, a series of infant illnesses, withdrawal of medications, and weaning from the apnea monitor. All interventions were successful, and no hospitalizations were needed.

The NCM also taught the family about infant nutrition, behavior, growth, and development of premature babies. She helped the family obtain developmental screening for the infants and helped the four-year-old sibling adjust to the new babies. Many times, the mother called the NCM for advice before calling the primary care physician. This sometimes eliminated a call to the physician; however, the mother also learned when to go directly to the clinic for medical interventions.

The NCM believes this family views her as a nurse and a family friend. She has been invited to the older sibling's dance programs and most recently to the twins' first birthday party, where she was introduced as "the girls' nurse."

Benefits of Nurse Case Management

There are recurring themes of partnering in caring as nurse case managers tell their stories about their clients and families. Clients refer to the NCM as "my nurse." Physicians and other members of the health care team call these nurses skilled patient advocates who provide a valuable service to the patient and family by communicating clinically relevant information in a timely manner. The physicians also note that coordinated care for complex patients by NCMs results in enhanced clinical and financial outcomes.

Changes in resource utilization are evident. Average lengths of stay decrease when NCM clients are hospitalized. There are fewer hospital admissions, and there is a longer time span between the admissions. Satisfaction surveys of clients having an NCM are very positive. The clients indicate that they no longer feel so alone with their illness or health problem.

Integrated Information Infrastructure

Providing continuity of care from one setting or provider to another requires efficacious use of communication technology. The separate information systems currently in use do not allow for transfer and exchange of information. Even when computer systems are in place, the mechanisms to exchange databases are often unavailable. An integrated system requires an electronic clinical record that inputs data into a central repository with a master patient index. Evaluating the effectiveness of the continuum of care is dependent on the analysis of interventions and outcomes, which can be supported only by an integrated information infrastructure.

Computer technology will only take us so far. We will need to have a standardized language to measure interventions and outcomes. The computer can retrieve and present data, but the data must be in a common language. Consensus on the language needs to be reached prior to computerizing the communication process. It requires collaboration among the health care team to define a common vocabulary with a variety of dictionaries. The electronic medical record will span the care continuum and facilitate care over time and settings. Computer technology is vital to this process, but there also needs to be a shared vision and common guiding principles on which to base decisions. For instance, informatics specialists must understand the concepts of the care continuum and not be bound by the organizational structure and traditional functions such as billing, data entry, and patient registration.

Health care providers have been slow to recognize the powerful influence of home and community interventions on health behaviors. Attention is currently focused on what happens within the walls of hospitals, with little thought about what happens with patients and families in their living environments. A paradigm shift will occur as patients and families become empowered to take responsibility for their own health. Currently, someone else holds the information, shares some part of it, and then expects the patient and family to make an informed decision. Unfortunately, health care providers sometimes resort to coercion or a punitive approach in order to obtain a desired decision. If the patient and family controlled the information in collaboration with their health care partners, health care strategies could be discussed and mutually agreed upon. Health care providers must give up control over the patient's information and be willing to teach them what the information means and how to use it to maximize health potential throughout life.

Advances in computer technology will allow people to be as well informed as their health care providers. Interactive computer programs could replace home visits or office visits and allow patients to assess their own health status and contribute data to their health record. Consumers, patients, and families will be able to access disease management strategies. This information will be transformed into knowledge, which can influence behavior. The paradigm shift occurs when the knowledge is held by individuals and families in addition to the health care providers. For instance, the Internet will provide people with detailed listings of referral sources and disease processes at any time of the day or night.

Summary

Management of health issues among clients at risk and those with chronic disabilities will be addressed in the community setting. Acute episodic illness will be seen as a process in the continuum of care and not as a single event. Ethical decisions about the availability of care and entitlement to medical services will need to be addressed as the proportion of elderly in our society increases. Limited financial resources will force society to make hard decisions about who gets what. Technology has developed faster than the ability to make ethical decisions. Personal desire drives many decisions to pursue aggressive treatment or to sustain life. Emotions run high in grief situations and can preclude the ability to make a rational or intelligent decision. A balance of individualism, utilitarianism, and humanism must be reached before society can begin to address the issues of quality across the continuum of care and work together to build healthy communities.

REFERENCES

Bauer, J. (1998). *Not what the doctor ordered: How to end the medical monopoly in pursuit of managed care* (2nd Ed.). New York: McGraw-Hill.

Bringewatt, R. (1995). You have not yet begun to integrate. *Health Systems Review.* Sep–Oct, *28* (5): 50–54.

Cohen, E. L. (1996). *Nurse case management in the twenty-first century.* St. Louis, MO: Mosby.

Doran, K., Sampson, B., Staus, R., Ahern, C., & Schiro, D. (1997). Clinical pathway across tertiary and community care after an interventional cardiology procedure. *Journal of Cardiovascular Nursing, 11*(2): 1–14.

Goldsmith, J. C., Goran, M. J., & Nackel, J. G. (1995). Managed care comes of age. *Health Care Forum Journal, 38,* 14–20, 22–24.

Gordon, M. (1987). *Functional health patterns. Nursing diagnosis: Process and application.* New York: McGraw-Hill.

Hargrove, R. A. (1998). *Mastering the art of creative collaboration.* New York: McGraw Hill.

Langfitt, T. W. (1990). *Forward to healthy America: Practitioners for 2005.* Philadelphia, PA: Pew Charitable Trusts.

Martin, K. S., and Scheet, N. J. (1992). *The Omaha System: A pocket guide for community health nursing.* Philadelphia, PA: W.B. Saunders.

McBeth, A. & Weydt, A. (1996). Innovative delivery systems: Freedom, trust, caring. In E. L. Cohen, (Ed.). *Nurse case management in the twenty-first century.* p. 105. St. Louis, MO: Mosby.

Senge, P. M. (1990). *The fifth discipline: The art and practice of the learning organization.* New York: Doubleday Currency.

The Health Futures Institute (1993). *LifeHealth: Transferring our vision of health.* Conference Handout, October 1993. Minneapolis, MN: Health Futures Institute.

Winer, M. (1995). More than the sum of individuals—A case collaboration. *Creative Nursing 1*(1): 9–11, Sep–Oct.

CHAPTER

7 Quality Evaluation

DOUGLAS L. WOOD
MARY I. HUNTLEY
KAY HUBBARD

Quality is never an accident; it is always the result of high intentions, sincere effort, intelligent direction and skillful execution; it represents the wise choice of many alternatives.

—Willa R. Foster

- The Challenge of the Twenty-First Century
- Research and Evaluation Models
- Improving Quality
- Summary

Health care delivery in the United States is characterized by uneven utilization of resources and somewhat unpredictable risks (Hannan, Kilburn, Racz, Shields & Chassin, 1994; Wennberg, 1994; Leape et al., 1995). As resources for building healthy communities become more constrained, it will be important to develop and apply measures that can distinguish true quality differences among providers, hospitals, and health plans. Such measures should be easy for users to understand, easy to collect and report, and within regular budget guidelines for collection and use of the data.

There are major concerns about the overutilization of tests and procedures that occurs in fee-for-service medicine, and there are growing concerns about underutilization of diagnostic and therapeutic interventions in managed care systems (Wennberg, 1994). There is also some concern about abuse of tests and procedures. The outcomes achieved with the application of diagnostic and therapeutic interventions in symptomatic patients and the use of preventive measures in asymptomatic or minimally symptomatic patients are also under scrutiny. More specifically, payers are reluctant to reimburse for tests and procedures that do not provide value or that are not considered necessary and appropriate. Given these circumstances, purchasers and consumers are seeking measures of quality that can assist them in choice of providers (McGowan, Evans & Michl, 1995).

The science of quality evaluation is growing with the development of meaningful and economical quality evaluation systems. There is a critical need for patients, purchasers, payers, providers, and others to work and learn together as the science of quality evaluation is advanced into the next century.

The Challenge of the Twenty-First Century

The challenge for quality evaluation in the twenty-first century will be to transform billions of bits of data into useful information which can then be used to generate knowledge. This process requires critical evaluation of current practice, comparison of existing practice and available technology against new technology, and improvement in clinical processes and outcomes to achieve the best practice (see Figure 7.1).

Access to data is critical to success in clinical research, education, and improvement of practice (McGowan, Evans & Michl, 1995). Data must be obtained from the medical records of large numbers of patients to provide researchers with sufficient information to make inferences about nonmedical causes of specific disease states or outcomes. State and federal legislatures must make certain that unreasonable limits are not placed on researchers because of privacy concerns. The need of society to have such information outweighs the need to limit access to a patient's health record.

There is much emphasis on accountability and the management of outcomes. It must be emphasized that outcomes cannot be managed. Rather, the process of care is managed. Outcomes are the result of a complex interaction of biological, psychological, social, and spiritual factors that affect the behavior of an individual after an intervention by the health care delivery system. In many communities, poverty, lack of transportation, and language barriers prevent some people from accessing care. These

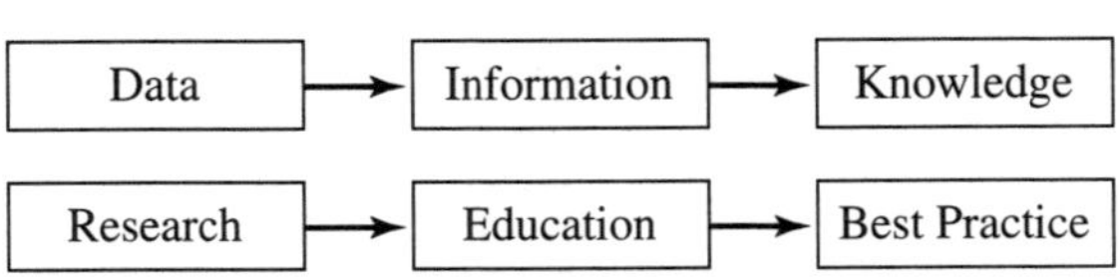

FIGURE 7.1 Quality Evaluation Information Flow Chart

Material taken from work completed through Immanuel St. Joseph's–Mayo Health System, Mankato, Minnesota, Office of Administration (1997). By permission.

social factors are often unknown to health care providers. Unfortunately, current quality evaluation methods are not sophisticated enough to determine the contribution of each of these factors to the ultimate outcome of a patient with a specific problem.

Larger scale, population-based studies will be necessary to understand the relationship of biological, psychological, social, spiritual, and medical interventions to certain outcomes. Studies of this scope will be more readily accomplished in health systems with (1) a large population base, (2) access to well-maintained medical records, (3) researchers (epidemiologists, data analysts, information systems specialists, and others), and (4) other resources to perform such studies.

It is important, however, to recognize that new relationships among purchasers, providers, and payers—and perhaps even government partnerships—could begin to provide researchers with access to larger patient populations and data resources. These relationships and resources could be used to carry out observational studies that would be of greater value to patients, payers, and policymakers. In a model used in Minnesota, physicians and an insurance company have entered into a working relationship in which physician groups participating in the insurance company's select cardiac network work collaboratively by using a common data collection instrument. The physician groups are responsible for reviewing the data and using the information to develop knowledge that can improve practice. For its part, the insurance company has agreed to provide financial support and to leave control over any published data to the physician groups. A similar model has been effective in northern New England (O'Connor et al., 1996).

Government partnerships have had some measure of success, although interagency disputes have presented a significant barrier. The Quality Assurance Reform Initiative (QARI), developed in 1991 and evaluated in a demonstration project in three states, is instructive. Aimed at Medicaid populations, QARI project results were mixed. Indeed, in states where health plans undertook internal efforts at quality improvement as part of the accreditation process with the National Committee for Quality Assurance, improvements in quality were greater than were demonstrated in the QARI project (Felt-Lisk & St. Peter, 1997).

Research and Evaluation Models

The methods of quality evaluation and research that will be required in the twenty-first century are diverse. Consumers of health care, whether they are well or ill at the time they make a purchasing decision or a decision about a diagnostic or therapeutic intervention, will have entirely different needs for information than payers, politicians, and policymakers. Patients who are ill with a significant, perhaps life-threatening, condition will have an entirely different perspective about what is important in terms of the quality of their interaction with health care providers and the skill of those providers than will their employer or insurer. As such, it must be recognized that the definition of quality and the description of desirable characteristics of a health care delivery system will vary according to the perspective of the person or organization asked to make a quality distinction.

Another vexing problem with design and implementation of quality evaluation and research is that of accountability. There is a growing effort to be able to assign accountability for outcomes to a specific physician, hospital, or health plan. As stated earlier, outcomes cannot be managed, but instead represent a complex interplay of variables and patient-related decisions.

Patients are often more concerned about access to care, availability of services, and the communication skills of physicians or other providers than about technical aspects of clinical care or clinical quality. They may be more inclined to make choices about a physician, surgeon, hospital, or health plan on the basis of information obtained from a friend or family member than on the basis of information from some other expert, their employer, a report card, the government, or media sources. Patients also seek information about how health plans, physicians, or hospitals care for patients who are ill, rather than information about utilization rates.

Patients also find it more difficult to evaluate clinical quality. Furthermore, the patient definition of quality differs from that of the clinician or surgeon as well as from that of the purchaser and payer. For example, a report card on a surgeon may indicate that the mortality of coronary bypass surgery in a particular hospital known to the patient is 3 percent, but another surgeon (unknown to the patient) in a renowned hospital ninety miles away has a mortality rate of 0.5 percent. Though the patient's insurer has determined that the second surgeon and hospital are the preferable providers, the patient wants surgery by a surgeon and hospital closer to home, where the patient is more comfortable with the providers. To the patients, the difference in mortality is simply not large enough to choose a more highly rated provider. Although experience from states where such programs have been in place suggests that surgical practices change when report cards are available (Hannan, Siu, Kumar, Kilburn & Chassin, 1995; Pennsylvania Health Care Cost Containment Council, 1995), it is not possible to determine, given our current tools, whether the improvement in outcome is a reflection of better surgical practice, better patient selection of surgeon, or some other factor. None of our current outcome measurement systems incorporate patient choice into the measurement tools.

The payer or purchaser is more interested in the appropriateness of the expenditure of dollars for interventions, but again the issues of quality measurement and accountability can be perplexing. Consider a sixty-five year old man with three-vessel coronary artery disease and impaired ventricular function who is also an insulin-dependent diabetic. Results from a large randomized trial of angioplasty and bypass surgery patients demonstrate that the mortality of patients with diabetes is much higher when angioplasty is chosen as treatment than when surgery is chosen, although the expense of uncomplicated angioplasty is considerably lower than the cost of bypass surgery (Bypass Angioplasty Revascularization Investigation, 1996; Hlatky et al., 1997). The patient is duly informed of these facts and decides that angioplasty is preferred. The cardiologist caring for the patient proceeds with angioplasty according to the patient's desires, but the patient dies after a procedural failure resulting in a fatal heart attack. The cardiologist made the right recommendation, but the patient overruled it, and the outcome was poor. The data collected will demonstrate a periprocedural complication and death, and perhaps an inappropriate angioplasty. Who is responsible for the poor outcome? No current quality measurement system has an effective method to account for patient choice or social factors in outcomes.

Consider the circumstance of a patient with coronary artery disease and high blood cholesterol. An expensive, highly effective cholesterol-lowering drug is prescribed, but the patient cannot afford the drug and does not have insurance coverage. The patient does not fill the prescription and has a fatal heart attack several months later. Who is responsible for the outcome? The physician made an appropriate clinical judgment, but the outcome was poor. The death may be ascribed to the physician as a failure of therapy. However, the real issue may be the design of the insurance package or the unwillingness of the government to provide resources for an underinsured individual.

These examples demonstrate very real problems that confront patients, purchasers, and policymakers in carrying out meaningful quality evaluations of providers and health plans, or that accurately ascribe an outcome to a medical intervention, patient choice, or a social or governmental cause. Quality measurement and research methods of the twenty-first century must address these and other problems of assignment of accountability.

The measures of quality must accurately discern true differences in outcomes based on the underlying health condition and related conditions, the treatment decisions of physicians, the decisions of patients, and the social factors that might influence outcome. These measures should incorporate the best available research findings on the management of the condition. The measures should be easy to obtain, and they must be reported to all involved so as to improve the likelihood that changes in care can improve outcomes. Health policy needs to ensure that the overall cost to obtain and report the information will not add significant administrative overhead expense, yet will provide information of benefit to all. The cost for a small physician practice to employ a person and acquire computer hardware and software to report outcomes may be thousands of dollars a year and would reduce the number of dollars that might be available for other programs, including patient care or community programs. For example, in the Mayo Health System, annual expenses for implementation of disease management strategies in a small practice (fewer than five physicians) are capped. The expenses for development of hardware and software needed for performance measurement are borne by the system rather than individual practices.

Resources to support quality measurement should come from all stakeholders. Insurers, purchasers, health plans, and government payers should also be willing to collaboratively devote resources to quality evaluation activities. This contribution may be in the form of a per case or per patient payment. Another alternative could be to consolidate the significant information system resources of payers as a foundation for continuing quality evaluation. Patients, providers, and others may then purchase the information resources needed to carry out quality evaluation and improvement activities. Purchasers and providers should also support quality measurement and evaluation as well as population measures and technology assessment activities by devoting a portion of the per employee contribution to such activities. The Institute for Clinical Systems Integration (ICSI), developed in 1992 by the Group Care Consortium in response to the first contract with the Buyers' Health Care Action Group, a consortium of self-insured businesses in the Minneapolis–St. Paul region, is a good model (HealthPartners, Park Nicollet Clinic & the Mayo Clinic, 1992). Business representatives serve on consortium committees, such as the committee responsible for the development, implementation, and measurement of performance of clinical guidelines (see Appendix D) and the technology assessment committee, which is responsible for assessing application of newer technologies in patient care and developing recommendations for technology utilization and payment policy.

Funding for large collaborative research projects must also be available from government, foundations, and private sources. The resources of the Agency for Health Care Policy and Research, the National Institutes of Health, and many other funding sources have been stretched by budget reductions. It will be necessary to seek new sources of funding and to reprioritize research efforts in order to best utilize existing dollars. Additionally, states and other governmental units that collect administrative data should make these data available for analysis and study. Improved communication and direct access to clinical and administrative data can reduce the cost of obtaining and analyzing data. The Internet provides cross-organizational communication that is inexpensive, widely available, and easy to use. Thus, states with wide area networks that could be made available for quality measurement and evaluation may find additional opportunities to reduce the cost of use of data.

As advances in regional networking reduce costs and barriers to effective utilization of large amounts of data are overcome, more political barriers to effective use of such information can be expected. Also, as more hospitals and clinics are merged into large corporate systems, sharing of information between systems becomes more limited.

A principal concern is confidentiality of administrative and health record data. Protection of confidentiality of health records can have unintended economic consequences for providers and health researchers as well as serious adverse effects on medical research. For example, the state of Minnesota recently adopted a patient medical record law that threatened the ability of epidemiologists and other researchers to gain access to a sufficient number of records to make statistically significant observations. The way the law was written and interpreted, if patients had not given written authorization indicating their consent for the use of information in their record, the record could not be used in epidemiological research. In the implementation of the statute, only 4 percent of patients at the Mayo Clinic refused to authorize use of their records, but 40 percent did not answer the question at all. This level of response, even after aggressive efforts to educate patients about the value of research, would make any study unreliable and difficult.

The Minnesota statute also required many steps to obtain authorization from patients to use the information in their records. At the Mayo Clinic, the initial costs to implement changes in registration and to set up information systems and the tracking systems required by the statute totaled almost two million dollars, and annual maintenance costs were estimated to exceed a half million dollars. The additional expense involved in such compliance creates an unnecessary burden for patients, providers, and society.

Improving Quality

The foregoing discussion suggests that the efforts to measure and improve quality in the health care system will yield limited results. There can be no question that an integral part of the delivery of health care is to organize quality evaluation and clinical research that will lead to better, more informed decisions. As a result of quality evaluation studies, an understanding of what works in health care, which treatments are most effective, which delivery systems are most efficient, how well clients are satisfied with their care, and how society can improve the health of populations will emerge.

The science of quality measurement is in its infancy, and there is a need for new and better measures. Such efforts are under way at the Foundation for Accountability, the Joint Commission for Accreditation of Health Care Organizations, the Agency for Health Care Policy and Research, the National Committee for Quality Assurance, and other organizations.

Patients, payers, and providers in hospital and community settings must apply available measures to current systems and work together to understand the implications of the results. By taking stock of the effectiveness of the measures and making appropriate changes, better measures can be developed and better results can be achieved. Shared accountability is needed to advance the science of quality measurement and the art of quality evaluation that are utilized making choices about health care. Otherwise, the pace of progress will be slowed unnecessarily. Until there are perfect quality measures, it is important to use available resources, such as the surveys and data available from county, state, and national sources, as the basis of future improvement efforts.

Some basic principles should govern future efforts at developing and using quality measures in health care. First, quality evaluation must be easy to use if it is to be successful and helpful to patients, payers, purchasers, policymakers, and the delivery system.

Second, the evaluation of quality should yield the knowledge needed to accomplish improvements in care. Otherwise, efforts at developing better quality measures are vulnerable to criticism and attack by all parties, and no progress will be made.

Third, it is critical to begin a cooperative effort that will help all stakeholders learn more about how quality evaluation should be used to serve multiple purposes. It will be important to develop better relationships between patients, payers, purchasers, providers, governments, and others. Strong leadership will be necessary from every group in order to develop the atmosphere of trust that will be critical to success.

Fourth, all sectors should be committed to an effort to reduce administrative costs and to use the savings to finance future development of information systems and other infrastructures to support the quality measurement and evaluation endeavor. This approach should also emphasize the need to develop networking that will permit better use of existing data resources and computer systems. Partnerships with universities, health services researchers, and others providing analytic skills should be undertaken to increase the likelihood of obtaining the requisite knowledge to improve practice.

Fifth, the overall effort should be economical in the choice of measures that can be readily implemented and understood by all users. Systems must be flexible to allow incorporation of new measures with a minimum of disruption of ongoing measurement efforts. The same flexibility should be pursued in use of hardware and software to support these efforts.

Finally, careful consideration of methods to maintain privacy of information obtained from health records will be important in earning the trust of consumers so that they will allow the use of health records in a positive, productive manner. Legislation proposed to produce confidentiality of medical information must be carefully crafted so as not to make analysis of medical information difficult or impossible—or excessively expensive to perform.

Summary

The need for excellent evaluation methods and tools in health care has never been greater, but the risks may never have been larger. Success will depend on cooperative efforts to advance a young science and develop the knowledge needed to improve our current practices and delivery systems. Shared accountability to develop such measures will be more important than accountability of individuals or organizations as we move into the twenty-first century. Healthy people and healthy communities depend on the collaborative, sincere, and skillful wisdom of many players working together. Quality cannot be left to chance.

REFERENCES

Bartlett, J. (1992). *Familiar quotations: A collection of passages, phrases, and proverbs.* Boston: Little & Brown.

Bypass Angioplasty Revascularization Investigation (BARI) Investigators. (1996). Comparison of coronary bypass surgery with angioplasty in patients with multivessel disease. *New England Journal of Medicine, 335,* 217–225.

Eddy D. (1997). Balancing cost and quality in fee-for-service versus managed care. *Health Affairs, 16,* 162–173.

Felt-Lisk, S. & St. Peter R. (1997). Quality assurance for Medicaid managed care. *Health Affairs. 16,* 248–252.

Hannan E. L., Kilburn, H., Jr., Racz, M., Shields, E., & Chassin, M. R. (1994). Improving the outcomes of coronary artery bypass surgery in New York State. *Journal of the American Medical Association, 271,* 761–766.

Hannan E. L., Siu, A. L., Kumar, D., Kilburn, H., Jr., & Chassin, M. R. (1995). The decline in coronary artery bypass graft surgery mortality in New York State: The role of surgeon volume. *Journal of the American Medical Association, 273,* 209–213.

Hlatky M. A., Rogers, W. J., Johnstone, I. Boothroyd, D., Brooks, M. M., Pitt, B., Reeder, G., Ryan, T., Smith, H., Whitlow, P., Wiens, R., & Mark, D. B. (1997). Medical care costs and quality of life after randomization to coronary angioplasty or coronary bypass surgery. *New England Journal of Medicine, 336,* 92–99.

Institute for Clinical Systems Integration (ICSI). (1992). Institute for Clinical Systems Guidelines, Bloomington, MN.

Leape, L. L., Bates, D. W., Cullen, D. J., Cooper, J., Demonaco, H. J., Gallivan, T., Hallisey, R., Ives, J., Laird, N., Laffel, G., et al. (1995). Systems analysis of adverse drug events. *Journal of the American Medical Association, 274,* 35–43.

McGowan, J., Evans, J., & Michl, K. (1995). Networking a need: A cost-effective approach to statewide health information delivery. In *Proceedings—The annual symposium on computer applications in medical care.* American Medical Informatics Association. Philadelphia, PA: 571–575

O'Connor, G. T., Plume, S. K., Olmstead, E. M., Morton, J. R., Maloney, C. T., Nugent, W. C., Hernandez, F., Jr., Clough, R., Leavitt, B. J., Coffin, L. H., Marrin, C. A., Wennberg, D., Birkmeyer, J. D., Charlesworth, D. C., Malenka, D. J., Quinton, H. B., & Kasper, J. F. (1996). A regional intervention to improve the hospital mortality associated with coronary artery bypass graft surgery. *Journal of the American Medical Association 275,* 841–846.

Pennsylvania Health Care Cost Containment Council. (1995). *A consumer guide to coronary artery bypass graft surgery, Volume IV: 1993 Data, June 1995.* Harrisburg, PA.

Wennberg, J. (1994). Dealing with medical practice variations: A proposal for action. *Health Affairs 8,* 6–32.

CHAPTER

8 Service–Education Partnerships

MARY KAY HOHENSTEIN
MARY I. HUNTLEY
SHARON P. AADALEN

A learning organization is an organization that continually expands its ability to shape the future.

—Peter M. Senge

- Theoretical Perspectives
  —Cultural Transformation Theory
  —Interorganizational Network Formation Theory
  —Social Change Theory
- Service–Education Partnerships Model
  —Horizontal Axis
  —Vertical Axis
- Case Studies
  —Regional Health Profile
  —Business and Industry Internship Program
  —Education–Service Partnership Council
  —Global Wireless Education Consortium
  —Regional Continuing Healthcare Education Center
- Summary

The vocabulary used in the literature of business (including the health care industry) and education (including schools of medicine and other health care providers) reflects the mental models that exist. Reference is made to "reengineering" our organizations (Griffith, Sahney & Mohr, 1995; Hammer & Champy, 1993). Patients are labeled "compliant" and "noncompliant." Medical care is assumed to be the same as health care, and the costs of both are said to be increasing (Halvorson, 1997). There are "managed care products," which are based on "capitation."

A term that will have increasing importance in the twenty-first century is *partnerships.* Partnerships of service, education, consumers, business, payers, legislators, and other organizational, institutional, and community leaders may provide the key to future healthy communities composed of healthy individuals (Eng, 1993).

Partnerships involve the establishment of mutually beneficial relationships. In order for partnerships to flourish, each partner needs to value the contributions and potential of the other. As in any joint endeavor, trust is essential. Are the people who work in health care agencies, institutions, and communities trusted to create their future, or is there need to control them? Is there careful listening to health care consumers and their families, acknowledging their expertise about their health care status and courses of actions, or is there authoritative prescribing and judging of client behavior related to outcomes? Are students heard when they express their desire to learn not only the knowledge and skills needed to provide care today but also information about future directions in health care?

Theoretical Perspectives

Three theoretical perspectives are relevant to the development of partnerships. They are cultural transformation theory, interorganizational network formation theory, and social change theory.

Cultural Transformation Theory

Cultural transformation theory was advanced by Eisler's research, which drew on art, archaeology, religion, social science, history, and other fields (Eisler, 1987). This theory proposes that the seeming diversity of human culture is undergirded by two basic social models: a dominator model and a partnership model. Dominator models rank human members in patriarchies and matriarchies, whereas partnership models are grounded in the principle of linking rather than ranking. Cultural transformation theory suggests that the earliest human cultures were relational, linking partnership models, not hierarchical dominator models. Table 8.1 compares dominator and partnership models, demonstrating prominent components of each.

Interorganizational Network Formation Theory

New knowledge and new technologies are mandating innovative interorganizational structures and strategies for coordinating complex human services (Alter & Hage, 1993). Interorganizational network formation theory is helpful in understanding similarities and differences of new self-organizing coalitions and partnerships, many of

TABLE 8.1 Comparison of the Three Basic Components of the Dominator and the Partnership Models

Component	Dominator	Partnership
Gender Relations	The ranking of the male over the female, as well as the higher valuing of the traits and social values stereotypically associated with "masculinity" rather than "femininity." (1)	Equal valuing of the sexes as well as of "femininity" and "masculinity," or a sexually egalitarian social and ideological structure.
Violence	A high degree of institutionalized social violence, including wife beating, rape, and warfare, with violence a structural component of the system.	A low degree of social violence, including wife beating, rape, and warfare, not a structural component of the system.
Social Structure	A generally hierarchic (2) and authoritarian social organization, with the degree of authoritarianism and hierarchism roughly corresponding to the degree of male dominance.	A generally egalitarian social structure.

Note.

(1) Reference here is to the dominator stereotypes of masculinity (associates "real men" with aggression, heroic violence, lack of feeling, and other "hard" traits) and femininity (associates women with soft traits such as caring, nonviolence, and compassion).

(2) Reference here is to the domination hierarchy under which social organization is maintained through force or the threat of force. The dominator form of hierarchy is contrasted with the actualization hierarchy (e.g., molecules, cells, and organs form higher, more complex, higher functioning subsystems of the human body).

From *The Partnership Way: New Tools for Living and Learning,* by R. Eisler and D. Loye (1998). Brandon, VT: Holistic Education Press, pp. 163–164. By permission of the authors.

which are service–education partnerships. Figure 8.1 illustrates three stages of network formation. The horizontal bar represents a continuum from embryonic exchange networks to fully developed systemic networks.

Network formation can be initiated at any of the stages. Development may be progressive, moving from stage 1 through stage 2 to stage 3, but it may also be nonlinear or cyclical. A coalition or partnership may emerge from a given stage and remain at that stage as it matures.

Katz and Kahn (1966) use the term *boundary spanners* to refer to individuals who actively initiate interorganizational networking with persons from other organizations

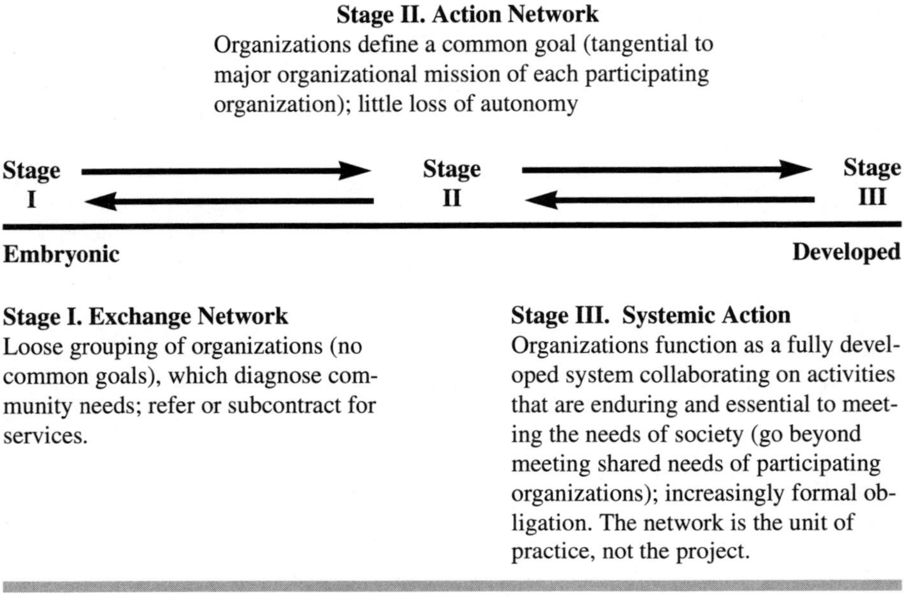

FIGURE 8.1 Three Stages of Network Formation

From Alter, C., Hage, J. (1993). *Organizations Working Together.* Newbury Park, Sage Publications. By permission of the publisher.

or institutions. Boundary spanners usually make contacts based on friendships, personal interest, self-development needs, and collegiality. There may be informal information exchange of technical information, tips on referrals, or sharing about continuing learning opportunities. When boundary spanners identify needed resources, they try to obtain them through the evolving interorganizational network.

There is no predetermined amount of time needed for network development. The length of time a network has been formed does not necessarily reflect the network's developmental stage. For service–education partnerships, integration of organizational participants is critical to assure continuous, dynamic, and dyadic informing of education by practice, and of practice by education.

A sense of identity differentiates networks at different stages of development. At stages 1 and 2, participants consider the network to be the sum of the participating organizations, and each participating organization retains significant autonomy. At stage 3, participating organizations function as a fully developed system in which the network is the unit of practice. A new system has formed in which the whole is greater than the sum of its parts. Cultural transformation theory suggests that life-giving cultural forms arise from models of social organization that are noncoercive and that value diversity.

Social Change Theory

Social change theory assumes that dominator forms of social organization result in poverty and discrimination and create unhealthy communities. Social change researchers have demonstrated the importance of studying strengths, assets, and resources in any community assessment. Further, they have demonstrated that environmental improvements that allow individuals to seek and fulfill their potential contribute to the health of the community. This theory is contrasted to social control theory, which emphasizes problems, needs, and weaknesses that are diagnosed and addressed by health and medical professionals.

Service–Education Partnerships Model

The service–education partnerships model evolved from the Health Bond experience (see Appendix A) as the participants had the opportunity to create and participate in building partnerships. Key concepts derived from the theories presented earlier and from experiences in a service–education partnership facilitated the creation of the model illustrated in Figure 8.2.

Each of the key concepts, represented by the four intersecting circles in Figure 8.2, has subconcepts that identify important features. At the intersection points of the circles are activities that generate the outcomes of a service–education partnership. The core concept of the model is the partnership itself. The horizontal axis names the kind of partnership—in this case, a service–education partnership. The vertical axis illustrates that the partnership begins with a mutual need or goal and generates agreed-upon outcomes for the customers it serves. All elements together are intended to represent an inclusive model that can help organizations develop a partnership.

The interactive planning concept was originally developed by Russell Ackoff (see Chapter 2). Associated with this concept are the subconcepts of vision, reality, stakeholders, research, and evaluation. Planning is based on a vision of where the partnership is headed. It acknowledges the reality of current health care. The principle of creative tension emerges when the partnership strives to reach the vision while attending to the dynamics of a real world and its stakeholders. Interactive planning must attend to the research data available and to what research needs to be done. Evaluation is a constant activity of the planning process. Data from consumer and community-based stakeholders, from the health care disciplines, and from market trends all play a role in planning and decisions made by the partnership for the community's health.

The second key concept in the model is interdisciplinary participants. Perspectives of a variety of disciplines help reduce duplication of services, improve communication, and assure that the best ideas from all perspectives are represented. The subconcepts depict the importance of a variety of talents and expertise that is essential

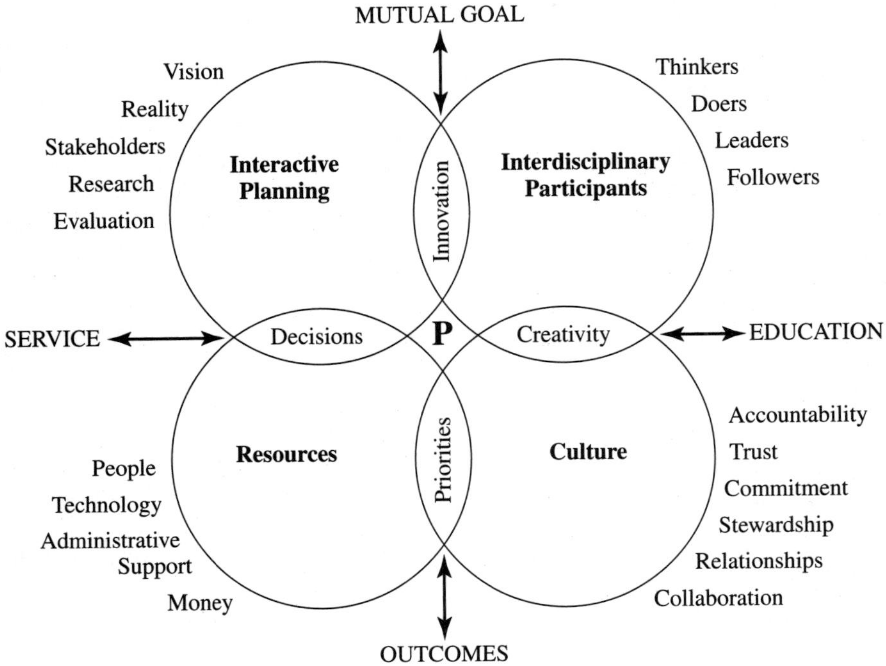

FIGURE 8.2 Service–Education Partnerships Model
From material developed by M. I. Huntley, M. K. Hohenstein, and S. P. Aadalen (1998). Mankato, MN. By permission.

to the partnership. The partnership needs people who are critical and reflective thinkers. It needs leaders, followers, and doers. All are active participants in the partnership, rather than passive observers. It is important for diversity to be represented in the partnership so that different disciplines and perspectives have a voice. From diversity comes creativity.

Culture, the third key concept, refers to the environment in which the partnership exists. The culture needs to be one in which the partners have a trusting relationship. Stewardship is valued and affirmed. Commitment is present. There is accountability to one another and to the partnership. Relationships are honest and respectful, and participants value the expertise each brings to the partnership. Communication is open; people feel listened to and cared about. There is collaboration over issues of importance to arrive at a consensus. In such a culture, the environment is seen as dynamic, created by the partnership itself and strengthened by the evolution of the partnership. The outcome is that the partnership is not only a way of doing business, but it is the right thing to do as well as the way to do things right.

Any partnership needs resources for its work. Resources include people to carry out the purposes and functions of the partnership, and money to support the goals.

Administrative support may provide leadership, empowerment, and encouragement to potential participants. Technology is necessary to facilitate effective use of other resources to achieve the partnership goals, for evaluation, and for creating expected outcomes. Technology includes computerized tracking of information and data, the use of multiple electronic systems, and so on. Partners may conduct meetings by interactive television or discuss important issues by electronic mail or Internet connections. A web page may be used to keep larger publics informed of the partnership's activities.

Interactive planning and resources come together when important decisions are made. Culture and resources help determine priorities. The interaction between culture and the interdisciplinary participants generates creativity. In a trusting environment, interactive planning with interdisciplinary participants leads to innovation. Decisions, priorities, creativity, and innovation are associated with all four key concepts. For example, decisions emerge not only from the interplay of the planning and resources but also as a result of the interplay of the interdisciplinary participants, culture, and resources. Often the decisions will be creative and innovative because of the interaction among the key concepts and the influence of the subconcepts. Likewise, priorities are determined not only from culture and resources but also as a result of the interactive planning process used by the interdisciplinary participants.

Partnership, the big *P* in the center of the model, is the core concept. The key concepts, subconcepts, and intersecting concepts together form a partnership. The partnership relationship experienced through Health Bond (Aadalen, 1996) was created through a grant initiative and became very highly valued. In fact, it was so highly valued that no one wanted it to end. Many discussions of how to continue the partnership were held as the grant project was nearing completion of its goal. The result is that new partnerships have formed. These partnerships are being valued in the same way because the important features represented in the model are present.

Horizontal Axis

On the horizontal axis of Figure 8.2 is the name of the partnership. It is easiest to explain a service–education partnership by examples. The examples described later in this chapter illustrate bringing people together from the domains of service, business or industry, and education. Education can be a system, a consortium of educational institutions, or individual colleges or universities. In the following examples, education partners were brought together from a technical college and a state university. Both institutions have autonomy of mission and purpose, although they are part of the same larger system within the state. What is important about a service–education partnership is that it is also the best way to attend to the mission and vision of respective organizations. In the dynamic age of information and technology, the partnership is an effective way to stay current in knowing how to best educate people for the workforce of today and tomorrow.

Vertical Axis

A mutual goal or need forms one side of the vertical axis in Figure 8.2. The goal of preparing the workforce of today and tomorrow is an example of a mutual goal shared by each of the partners and is a strong motivator to creating such a partnership. The work of the partnership to address the mutual goal or need then generates outcomes, which can be the measure of the success of the partnership. Strategies to measure and evaluate outcomes is a necessary function of the partnership. The outcomes provide evidence that the commitment of people and partners is valued and meaningful. Goals are accomplished, outcomes are valued, and the partnership continues to develop.

Case Studies

Five case studies demonstrate how the service–education partnership model has been applied. These initiatives were all directly or indirectly related to the activities of Health Bond (see Appendix A). They reflect varying amounts of cultural transformation, interorganizational networks, and social change. In each case, the partnerships developed have strengthened both service and education.

Regional Health Profile

Region Nine is a nine-county area in south-central Minnesota. It is a rural area with one city, Mankato, that is the regional center for the surrounding cities, towns, and farms. There are many health care organizations, education systems, businesses, and successful farms in this rich agricultural area. The area has a well-functioning regional government agency, the Region Nine Development Commission, that assists with collaborative projects to promote progress and enhance the quality of life for persons residing within the area.

The Regional Health Profile (RHP, 1994) was developed in response to the Healthy People 2000 national health and disease prevention objectives. It was a collaborative project involving each of the hospitals and county public health agencies in the nine-county area as well as Minnesota State University, Mankato, South Central Emergency Medical Services, and Region Nine's Area Agency on Aging and Community Drug Prevention Project. Each member agency contributed five hundred dollars, and Immanuel St. Joseph's–Mayo Health System underwrote and coordinated the project. Volunteers from each member organization provided the human resources for guiding this collaborative project.

Objectives included identifying regional health problems, establishing health priorities, facilitating collaborative planning in the region, and providing baseline information for comparison with future projects. The profile was based on a survey of health behaviors sent out to twenty thousand households across Region Nine during

1994. Respondents were asked questions about their ability to access and afford health care, their health habits, and their participation in screening tests and regular examinations. The response rate was approximately 30 percent.

The information gathered in the survey was used in projects, and members from participating organizations met to share information on the projects they were working on. A newsletter conveyed survey data results to project sponsors. A collaborative research effort within Region Nine resulted in local and regional projects addressing key health status indicators. Some of the projects were

- Implementation of the Minnesota Breast and Cervical Cancer Control Program
- Tobacco, alcohol, and substance abuse education
- Immunization promotion and special free or low-cost clinics
- Healthy Families Program aimed at children of overburdened families
- Teen pregnancy prevention
- Alternatives to nursing home care
- Depression screening for senior citizens, with follow-up seminar
- Domestic violence advocacy training program
- ENCARE (Emergency Nurses Cancel Alcohol Related Emergencies)

The research data from RHP has been utilized by Minnesota State University, Mankato, and South Central Technical College in curriculum development in nursing and allied health. Both institutions are major sources for regional health care providers. The outcomes were so successful that in 1998, twenty-seven county public health departments joined forces to conduct a follow-up profile and have obtained substantial financial support from health care providers.

Business and Industry Internship Program

Technical college instructors need to maintain current theory and skill levels for the occupational programs they teach. Knowing what is happening in business and industry can mean success or failure for graduates of occupational education programs. To make sure faculty members stay current, the Minnesota State Colleges and Universities System (MnSCU) has established an internship program for instructors in the technical colleges. This Business and Industry Internship Program is a staff development activity that relies on partnerships with organizations to provide work experiences in settings related to teaching assignments. In this program, MnSCU technical college faculty work full time for between three and six weeks in preapproved settings. The internship allows participants to validate their present skills and update and acquire new skills and thought processes.

Upon completion of the internship, participants add their new skills and knowledge to the curriculum, evaluate the internship program and site, and communicate with the site sponsor. The currency and relevancy of instruction supported by the

Business and Industry Internship Program may be in part responsible for Minnesota's reputation as a national leader in technical education.

South Central Technical College nursing and allied health program staff participate regularly in the internship program. Clinical site support is excellent from area health care organizations. This service-education partnership has enhanced relationships between institutions and improved communication among clinical staff and faculty members.

Education–Service Partnership Council

What knowledge, concepts, strategies, and skills do nurses need in the twenty-first century? This question has been asked in many health care and education institutions. Faculty representatives from Minnesota State University, Mankato, School of Nursing get together with leaders of community health care organizations to explore this and others questions at regular Education–Service Partnership Council meetings. A collaborative forum has been created in which members share ideas and perspectives about preparing the nursing workforce for the twenty-first century.

Partners have included the local hospital, a tertiary center, long-term care, home care, public/community health, spiritual care, and medical/primary care. Also serving on the council have been consumers, alumni, and students from undergraduate and graduate nursing programs.

The major goal of the Education–Service Partnership Council has been ongoing exchange of information about health care workforce needs and requirements, changes in educational curriculum, and learning opportunities. Topics include changes in health care; student, education program, and clinical agency successes and innovations; accreditations; faculty challenges and development; funding and grants; curriculum content; and organizational structure.

The council facilitated partnership infrastructure development, which has allowed maximal proaction as well as responsiveness of education and service to workforce demands. Council members want to develop the partnership so that it can make a difference in the preparation of tomorrow's nurse. To this end, the council has positioned itself to influence public policy and has received state funding to deal with such health care issues as recruitment, curriculum, and program delivery.

Global Wireless Education Consortium

The Global Wireless Educational Consortium (GWEC) began as a stage two network, halfway between embryonic and developed (see Figure 8.1). However, the commitment of substantive shared resources by all partners early in partnership formation made it possible for GWEC to move rapidly toward stage three, a system network with increasingly formalized relationships. All partners have committed to collaborating on essential needs related to the wireless industry and the preparation of a workforce to support the industry's development.

Minnesota State University, Mankato, and South Central Technical College have partnered with AT&T and several other wireless industry giants in a unique consortium aimed at educating new engineers and technicians for the rapidly growing wireless communications industry. The consortium headquarters is located at an industrial development corporation responsible for supporting business and industry in the Mankato area. Local business leaders have marketed Mankato and North Mankato as a national training site for the wireless industry in the hopes of attracting related businesses to the area:

> The cooperative agreement is a national model that is drawing attention from dozens of the top corporations involved in the cellular industry. AT&T, Minnesota State University, Mankato, South Central Technical College and others agreed to a partnership in which the schools would tailor programs for the advanced wireless communications training for AT&T workers. In exchange, AT&T and other companies will pay between $350,000 and $500,000 a year and provide equipment. (The Free Press, Mankato, February 20, 1997)

The partnership has been named the Institute for Wireless Education. Guest lecturers and industry experts work with educational partners to develop and improve existing curriculum and to turn out graduates with up-to-date knowledge and skills.

AT&T's competitors have been encouraged to join the consortium. This fast-growing industry wanted to avoid the kinds of problems that have plagued the computer industry. Sharing curriculum and developing a standardization process have helped avoid these pitfalls. Lucent Technologies, Ericksson (Motorola), and the University of Texas at Dallas have all joined the consortium.

The director of technical education at AT&T has stated that the presidents of Minnesota State University, Mankato, and South Central Technical College were willing to work with industry to develop the curriculum: "They're very progressive. It's very unique in the education world to find schools willing to do this. They stepped to the plate first." (*The Free Press,* Mankato, February 20, 1997)

Regional Continuing Healthcare Education Center

The Regional Continuing Healthcare Education Center (ReCHEC) exemplifies service–education partnerships in their truest form. This organization began with a small gathering of people who have turned wishful thinking into reality through commitment to vision, collaboration, inclusiveness, visionary thinking, and action for the quality of health care in south-central Minnesota.

ReCHEC began in 1993 at an informal meeting between two staff education members of Immanuel St. Joseph's–Mayo Health System, the director of continuing education from Minnesota State University, Mankato, School of Nursing, and the health coordinator of South Central Technical College. This meeting had been called to discuss what each organization was planning to do in nursing continuing education.

It could have been more appropriately titled the annual "turf protection" meeting. The usual discussion of needing better communication when scheduling conferences and workshops in order to keep attendance strong took place. The people involved knew each other well, and they trusted one another enough to honestly discuss the issues. Soon they were talking about what an ideal nursing continuing education model might look like for the region. Terms like stakeholders, cooperation, collaboration, trust, visioning, commitment, quality, and nursing center emerged. They realized that "something is really happening here," and they decided to keep meeting on a regular basis. Thus ReCHEC was born.

ReCHEC now consists of sixteen voluntary service and education organizations. Members have met monthly to fulfill the mission of providing "collaborative learning opportunities to enhance high quality care."

A comprehensive needs survey of RNs, LPNs, nursing assistants, home health aides, and allied health professionals from south-central Minnesota provided information for council members to complete continuing education planning. This survey and much of ReCHEC's early work was supported by Health Bond's Robert Wood Johnson Foundation/Pew Charitable Trusts grant to strengthen hospital nursing (Aadalen, 1996).

The Minnesota State Colleges and University System (MnSCU) awarded a $35,000 grant to ReCHEC in 1996 to support further development of the organization. The grant committee selected ReCHEC because of its strong partnership with area health care provider organizations. This is an example of how funding has followed service–education partnerships after they are formed, rather than using grant dollars to develop partnerships.

Council members attended national nursing technology conferences together to gain information on how best to offer continuing education to area health care providers. Other conference attendees have often commented on how unusual it is to see education and service members from the same location traveling together and working so collaboratively on a mutual project. ReCHEC members take this approach for granted.

Continuing education has been available to service organizations and individuals, at a reasonable cost, by accessing ReCHEC videotapes, CD-ROMs, and laptop computers through the technical college library. Items are sent to organizations or individuals for use at their facility or in their own home. Continuing education credit has been granted, upon request, by ReCHEC.

All resource materials have been listed in a directory distributed to south-central Minnesota service provider organizations and individuals. Additional resource materials are available through EduMed, a private company specializing in continuing education in radiology. A contract with EduMed has added educational resources in several delivery formats, which financially benefits both organizations. The Minnesota Area Geriatric Education Center, located at Minnesota State University, Mankato, has also contributed to the resource library.

ReCHEC has had solid support from Minnesota State University, Mankato, South Central Technical College, and area health care organizations. Indications that

ReCHEC has become a systemic network can be found in the partnership's name change. The last C in ReCHEC now stands for the word *Center,* rather than the word *Council* used originally. The potential for valuable projects has remained high due to its solid foundation as a service and education organization.

Summary

The partnership model can be used regardless of the developmental stage of the partnership. An important outcome of a service–education partnership is creation of quality, cost-effective, accessible education for practice in the work world. A mutual goal is often a driving force for the partnership to form. An outcome of forming the partnership is being able to position oneself to receive additional funding. The value of partnerships is more fully realized after the partnership is in place, as it is then that funding to support the partnership comes forth.

The goals of creating healthy people and healthy communities in the twenty-first century can be accomplished through service–education partnerships, providing the motivating mutual goal for service and educational organizations to create a partnership. The partnership model provides a framework organizations can use to make a difference in the lives of people and communities.

REFERENCES

Aadalen, S. P. (Ed). (1996). *Health Bond: Building opportunities new directions.* Mankato, MN: Health Bond.

Alter, C. & Hage, J. (1993). *Organizations working together.* Newbury Park, CA: Sage Publications.

Eisler, R. (1987). *The chalice and the blade.* San Francisco: Harper San Francisco.

Eisler, R. & Loye, D. (1990). *The partnership way.* San Francisco: Harper San Francisco.

Eng, E. E. (1993). Partnership theory. In *Proceedings: Nurse leadership: caring for the emerging majority: Empowering nurses through partnerships & coalitions.* Washington, D.C.: Division of Nursing, Bureau of Health Professions, Health Resources Administration; Office of Minority Health, Office of Assistant Secretary; and Department of Health & Human Services, Public Health Service.

Griffith, J. R., Sahney, V. K., & Mohr, R. A. (1995). *Reengineering health care: Building CQI.* Ann Arbor, MI: Health Administration Press.

Halvorson, G. C. (1997). Higher costs, but better care: Medical costs reflect improved treatments. *Minneapolis Star Tribune,* July 21, p. A9.

Hammer, M. & Champy, J. (1993). *Reengineering the corporation: A manifesto for business revolution.* New York: Harper Collins.

Katz, P. & Kahn, R. (1966). *The social psychology of organizations.* New York: John Wiley.

The Free Press, Mankato, MN (1997, February 20.).

Regional Health Profile (1994). Mankato, MN: Health Bond, Immanuel St. Joseph's Hospital, Region Nine Development Commission, and Minnesota State University, Mankato.

Senge, P. M. (1990). *The fifth discipline: The art and practice of the learning organization.* New York: Doubleday Currency.

CHAPTER

9 Building Healthy Communities

Unifying Health Care

KATHRYN D. SCHWEER

ANNETTE J. McBETH

The future belongs to those who believe in the beauty of their dreams.

—Eleanor Roosevelt

- Unifying Values
  - —Freedom and Responsibility
  - —Quality and Affordability
  - —Accessibility and Acceptability
  - —Assessment and Assurance
  - —Partnerships and Networking
  - —Integrity and Respect
  - —Compassionate Caring and Service Commitment
- Unifying Goals
  - —Vision of a Healthy Community
  - —Meeting Current Health Challenges
- Unifying Elements
- Unifying Tools
  - —Change
  - —Networking
  - —Leadership
  - —Information Technology
- Unifying Strategies
  - —Preventive Guidelines
  - —Complementary/Alternative Healing
  - —Collegial Collaboration
- Summary

What will health care be like in the twenty-first century? Will the current fragmented, illness-care-dominated system be perpetuated? Or will individual and community health needs—of mind, body, and spirit—be met in an atmosphere of mutual trust, respect, and choice?

The challenge ahead is to develop an integrated, holistic health system that serves people throughout the lifespan. A shared vision of health, based on common values and trust, will be needed, as will a paradigm shift away from the current system, which was designed and developed around the 10 percent of the population who are sick. Westberg (1990) advocates focusing on the other 90 percent of the population as we move forward.

Unifying Values

The predominant value of twentieth-century American health care was conquering disease. The system focused on medical diagnosis and treatment of illnesses. Major efforts succeeded in eliminating smallpox and greatly reducing the incidence of all infectious diseases. But despite these accomplishments, people and communities still face many health problems. Clearly a new focus on health is needed for the twenty-first century.

Values deemed important in order to achieve a health care delivery system include: freedom and responsibility, quality and affordability, accessibility and acceptability, assessment and assurance, partnerships and networking, integrity and respect, as well as compassionate caring and service commitment. Recommendations for fulfilling these values follow.

Freedom and Responsibility

- Allowing choices within an integrated system so that people decide how they want to work toward the goal of healthier individuals and communities
- Working with people in communities to develop individual responsibility for healthful behaviors.

Quality and Affordability

- Promoting culture change in health care organizations so that both providers and consumers are involved in achieving continuous quality improvement and cost containment
- Achieving high clinical quality standards and superior service throughout the care continuum, while being stewards of the available resources
- Addressing societal wishes for quality cost-effective care while facing the realities of economics, ethics, and resource limitations

- Designing outcome measurement systems built on continuous quality improvement principles that address customer satisfaction, clinical outcomes, and cost.

Accessibility and Acceptability

- Developing integrated health care delivery systems that can be accessed by all people throughout the life continuum
- Improving the process of care and performance through user-friendly information systems that incorporate meaningful measures that can be utilized by all consumers and providers.

Assessment and Assurance

- Assessing our communities and regions to determine ways to improve health status and to set standards and policies for public health issues
- Enhancing our successes in public health measures that have improved the quality of life and extended our lifespan, such as sanitation, communicable disease control, and environmental health
- Assuring that adequate attention and resources are focused on prevention of current threats to the community's health, such as AIDS, tuberculosis, *E. coli* in food, hepatitis C, and contaminated water supplies.

Partnerships and Networking

- Developing partnerships between public and private providers of health care, between education and service, and between caregivers and those receiving health care
- Involving all components of the community in determining the health care goals for the twenty-first century and in planning for the resources and methods to attain those goals
- Developing partnerships for research projects to test new approaches to alleviating root causes of poor health, such as poverty, crime, and violence
- Promoting networking within and between systems to overcome the inertia of "the way we have always done things."

Integrity and Respect

- Renewing confidence in the health care delivery system by being trustworthy in all interactions and by communicating openly, honestly, and responsibly
- Valuing the innate dignity and respecting the uniqueness of every person
- Recognizing the diversity of the people we serve and with whom we work
- Encouraging the development of each person's full potential.

Compassionate Caring and Service Commitment

- Affirming that caring and service are the essential elements of health care delivery
- Linking caring and service to the other values that guide our delivery of health care
- Finding new ways to acknowledge and reward excellence in compassionate caring and service so that people have a better understanding of their effect on building healthier communities:

> This is the ideal time to tackle problems in the health care system, to bring all players together, to put health first. It will be hard work. We have the knowledge, the tools, and the ability. But we must seek something short of Camelot, something that is sustainable. But considering what we have before us, it is an economic imperative. It is an ethical imperative. Press on. (Lewin, 1997, pp. 5–9)

Unifying Goals

Our future belongs to us. With unifying values to guide us, we can be the architects of the twenty-first century health care delivery system. Achievement of healthy people and healthy communities is the goal.

Vision of a Healthy Community

One vision of a healthy community includes the following: Every child is a wanted child. Family members nurture one another and provide a safe environment for learning values and life skills. Schools and parents work together to create places where children and adults thrive and engage in lifelong learning. Community resources for health, safety, transportation, arts, recreation, spiritual, and other needs are available and accessible to all. Elders are integrated into the life of the community in meaningful and productive ways. Basic needs for food, clothing, and shelter are met. Opportunities for satisfying work and economic growth are available to all.

Each person and each community will have different, but similar, visions of what a healthy community is. To attain the envisioned future, current health challenges must be met.

Meeting Current Health Challenges

Hancock and Garrett (1995) have stated that the current threats to health in industrialized countries are population growth, urbanization, environmental change, poverty, inequity, war, existing communicable and chronic diseases, and possible new diseases. They note that improvements in health over the past hundred and fifty years have primarily resulted from better economic, environmental, and social conditions, not from medical care:

> Stated quite simply, people cannot be well if they lack the basic prerequisites for good health. To be healthy, they must have decent housing, adequate nutrition, access to safe water and basic sanitation, a safe and non-toxic environment, and freedom from violence. They also must have means to support themselves economically, to participate politically in decisions about their own lives, and to obtain primary health care when necessary. Unless these basic needs are met, health is impossible, regardless of medical miracles and sophisticated health care systems. (Hancock & Garrett, 1995, p. 937)

Another challenge is the improper use of managed care. As a response to escalating health care costs, managed care approaches have been adopted nationwide. Suzanne Gordon, in her book *Life Support,* describes the situation as follows:

> In our uniquely American health care system, one that depends on private insurance provided as a benefit of employment—employers large or small are trying to save premium dollars by pushing employees into health maintenance organizations or other forms of managed care. (Gordon, 1997, p. 251)

According to Gordon, such practices as dictating choice of physician, gag clauses for health care providers, shortened lengths of hospital stay, and hospital restructuring or downsizing are having a devastating effect on the quality of care. It is clear that "America must deal with an utterly irrational health care financing system that allows private interests to make billions from the pain and suffering of their fellow citizens" (Gordon, 1997, p. 308).

Unifying Elements

The design for a healthy future for people and communities will have as its foundation six interactive planning elements.

Regionalization involves implementing a consumer-driven integrated health system that ensures choice within the constraints of finite resources to achieve improvement of the health status of the population and communities served.

Shared visioning means creating a mutually held goal of an integrated health care system, engaging community leaders and representative stakeholders, and utilizing the framework of Healthy People 2010 in order to achieve healthier people and healthier communities.

The *culture of health care* will need to undergo change from primary care to community primary health care. In order to build individual, community, and regional health, active partnerships that engage in self-management and accountability for health throughout the lifespan must be developed and implemented.

Continuum of care requires reengineering our present system away from diagnosis and treatment and toward community care management, utilizing incentives for individuals, families, and neighborhoods who take responsibility for their own health and well-being over the lifespan.

Quality evaluation requires deriving measures that accurately discern the true differences in outcomes based on the underlying health and related conditions, the treatment decisions of physicians, the decisions of patients, and the social factors that might influence outcomes.

Service–education partnerships establish frameworks for working together across systems. The synergism that results from joint efforts to prioritize and meet community health needs creates the potential for new and better health outcomes.

Unifying Tools

Several tools are available for use by those who are building healthy communities. Although resistance to change is pervasive, society is adapting to change whenever the change process is managed well. Networking is discussed briefly in this chapter and serves as a powerful tool which can lighten the load and make the building effort more interesting and satisfying. Sound leadership and wise use of information technology are additional tools that assist communities to meet their goal of becoming healthy places for people to live.

Change

Adapting to change on an individual, corporate, industry, national, and global level will be imperative for health care in the twenty-first century. Our structures will change to allow for more cooperation, collaboration, and flexibility as we meet changing priorities (Senge, Kleiner, Roberts, Ross, Roth, & Smith, 1999). Our operations will change as health care providers and consumers have different motivation and perspective on what needs to be done to improve the health of our people, communities, and world. Our strategies will include the latest technology as well as the shared values of caring and service.

Health care will change even more quickly in the twenty-first century than it did in the last few decades (Davis & Meyer, 1998). The knowledge explosion has not bypassed health care, and keeping up with the latest diagnostic and treatment modalities will continue to be a major challenge for providers and consumers alike. The only way to survive is to constantly try to find new and better ways of providing our services. Health care consumers and providers will need a positive attitude toward change, tolerance of ambiguity and uncertainty, and willingness to adapt.

Networking

By developing contacts and exchanging information with others, we are able to learn from one another, serve as resources to each other, and get support and assistance from many people. Heterick (1997) claims that most management theories have failed

> because they haven't understood or internalized the lessons of networking. The governing motivators of networking are not capital, or command and control, but rather diffused information and self-serving cooperation. (p. 1)

Networks of health care providers are being developed and will likely play a dominant role in the twenty-first century. Most managed care plans, such as health maintenance organizations and physician provider organizations, are networks of insurers, providers, and employers. Learning to work productively within these networks while maintaining core values will require new levels of cooperation by the entire health care team, the insurers, and the people receiving health care. Gordon (1997) has

> become convinced that the only victories we can win over our vulnerability and mortality are those of the human spirit and human community. Nurses and the patient relationships they forge create that kind of community. They not only help us to heal, they embody the more powerful and enduring victory of care. (p. 308)

Networks have a vital role in the acceptance of any new product or service. In his review of studies of the diffusion of innovation, Rogers (1983) noted the power of networks:

> Most individuals do not evaluate an innovation on the basis of scientific study of its consequences. Most depend mainly upon a subjective evaluation of an innovation that is conveyed to them from other individuals like themselves who have previously adopted the innovation. This dependence on the communicated experience of near-peers suggests that the heart of the diffusion process is the initiation by potential adopters of their network partners who have adopted previously. (p. 18)

Leadership

To achieve the goal of healthy people and healthy communities requires leaders who consistently ask, "How does this affect the client, family, neighborhood, community, or region?" Leadership is critical in articulating and modeling core values and in gathering resources for change. Health care organizations in the twenty-first century will require many leaders who are able to work together, involve the clients they serve, and create and maintain a shared vision of what needs to be done to make their communities healthier places to live. Such leaders will need to

- Be visionary
- Inspire and empower others
- Communicate effectively with all people, using all available communications methods
- Practice ethically and consistently

- Be sensitive to others' feelings and needs
- Take joy in the accomplishments of others and pride in the work of the group, rather than self-pride or self-importance
- Be master strategists in avoiding conflicts by dealing with problems or conflicts in a fair and timely manner
- Embrace and facilitate change

Information Technology

The technological innovation that has had the greatest effect on health care at the end of the twentieth century is the computer. All the other technology used in diagnosing and treating disease is dependent on computer support. The rapid dissemination of knowledge now possible through computer networks is changing the way health care providers and consumers interact, the way care is provided, and the management of and payment for care. In the twenty-first century, the need for specialized knowledge will grow, and the application of knowledge will result in new organizations and specialists. Handling all this information will require empowered employees capable of providing leadership in their sphere of activity and creatively working with others.

Information technology applications currently in use in business and industry will become the norm in health care delivery. An electronic health record, such as the master patient index described in Chapter 6, will probably be available early in the twenty-first century. The potential for improving clinical outcomes and service quality throughout the continuum of care, involving individuals in health care decisions, and analyzing the cost-effectiveness of care will be enhanced as information technology is utilized more fully.

Unifying Strategies

Building healthy communities requires the involvement of more than health care providers. An integrated health care delivery system is only one aspect. In the twenty-first century, the preventive guidelines already available will guide community efforts. Natural/alternative/complementary healing approaches will be tested and used by many people, whether or not they are recognized by mainstream health care providers. Full integration of the health care delivery system with community partners who are committed to their social responsibility for improving community health will provide the necessary force for building healthy communities.

Preventive Guidelines

Clinical guidelines, such as those of the Institute for Clinical Systems Integration (see Appendix D), use an interdisciplinary and evidence-based approach for both preventive services and disease screening. Pediatric guidelines target low-risk, asymptomatic children from birth to eighteen years of age. Adult guidelines are available for those aged nineteen and over. Generally, these guidelines do not address the needs of pregnant women or of individuals with chronic diseases or disorders. Interdisciplinary preventive service practitioners, including primary care physicians, nurse practitioners, physician assistants, and other clinical professionals with advanced training and education, are considered appropriate providers of preventive services.

Key implementation goals of the Institute for Clinical Systems Integration Guidelines (1994) are:

- Increasing the percentage of patients receiving appropriate preventive services as defined by their age- and sex-specific schedule recommendations
- Decreasing inappropriate tests administered at preventive care counseling visits
- Increasing the percentage of patients presenting themselves for preventive care who receive a health risk assessment

It is important to note that risk assessments occur at each preventive visit to identify risk factors that require counseling or special testing, such as substance abuse, nutrition, injury prevention, sexual practices, abuse and violence, and mental health awareness. Preventive health care guidelines help identify physiological conditions that interrelate with the emotional, social, and spiritual health of individuals and families.

Citizen groups play an essential role in preventive efforts. Community health education projects reach out to vulnerable groups. Programs promoting the use of seat belts and bicycle helmets and warning children about drug use have been successful in preventing accidents and drug abuse.

Complementary/Alternative Healing

For many decades, a small number of medical and health practitioners have espoused a more holistic approach to disease, illness, and health (Gottlieb, 1995). They have encouraged people to more actively participate in their own healing, to use complementary therapies, and to more fully incorporate mind and spirit into healing ventures.

The 1990s have seen an explosion of products, books, magazines, clinics, and practitioners devoted to holistic concepts (see, for example, Myss, 1996). Many health care forecasters believe that this movement will continue to accelerate into the twenty-first century as people have more access to information about multiple healing modalities.

The unifying values presented earlier in this chapter fit well with the movement toward complementary and alternative healing philosophies. *Freedom and responsibility* are the cornerstones of the holistic movement, allowing people to work with practitioners they choose. While *quality* needs to be more standardized, *affordability* is one of the most attractive features of holistic care. Although studies indicating that stress reduction for patients with heart disease can reduce their risk of having further heart problems by 75%, only about 10% of heart patients are offered information about stress reduction methods (Blumenthal et al., 1997). It is not difficult to calculate the amount of money saved if even 50% of heart patients had less risk of recurrence by using stress reduction modalities.

Other values are *accessibility and acceptability.* Studies indicate that even though insurance does not pay for most of the alternative care, more than a third of Americans visited alternative practitioners in the 1990s. Acceptability is very high, though finances continue to be a primary barrier.

The *partnership* model is at the core of the holistic movement. Not only are the practitioner and patient in partnership, but also there is continuing drive to bring in other support systems when necessary. These might include other practitioners (both conventional and alternative), case managers, spiritual mentors, relatives, educators, and other social support people. *Networking and collaborating* on an individual and system basis is the essence of holistic care.

Integration of our present system with the holistic model will be an important milestone for health care in the twenty-first century. Models of such integration include the Mind/Body Institute at Harvard University (Benson, 1979; Benson, 1996), The Center for Mind-Body Medicine, Washington, D.C. (Gordon, 1996), and the newly formed University of Minnesota Center for Spirituality and Healing (Kreitzer & Plotnikoff, 1997).

Collegial Collaboration

During the past century, modern medicine has taken the dominant role in decisions made about health care. Medical doctors not only diagnose and prescribe for individuals, but also determine how health care funds should be allocated. Organized medicine decides which diseases or treatments should be researched, which health care problems should be addressed, and which approaches should be tried. In order to move toward the goal of healthy people and healthy communities, medicine will have to shed its paternalistic models and work collaboratively with community leaders and other health care providers to assure that health care is available to all.

Primary care has traditionally meant medical care for acute episodes of illness. Third-party payers limited reimbursement for primary care to physicians until 1997, when amendments to the Omnibus Budget Reconciliation Act provided direct payment for advanced-practice nurses. Other third-party payers are also reimbursing care for health promotion, screening, chronic disease control, and management of common acute illnesses provided by nurse practitioners, clinical nurse specialists, and behavioral health providers. In some cases, complementary and alternative therapies are also eligible for third-party reimbursement.

A necessary first step toward collegial collaboration for community primary health care is the development of teamwork among physicians, nurses, and other allied health providers. Satinsky (1998) provides several exciting case examples of the positive results of an integrated care delivery system's focus on healthy communities.

Equally important is the active participation and collaboration of community residents if basic health care problems are to be resolved. Since 1989 the Search Institute in Minneapolis, Minnesota, has been engaged in a national effort to promote positive youth development focused on community collaboration among parents, adolescents, school, youth-serving agencies, congregations, and community leaders. Their research has uncovered forty assets young people need to develop to their full potential and to become productive citizens (Blyth, 1993).

As these examples illustrate, the involvement of the community is essential for building healthy communities. The role of health care professionals in the future is to enable people within the community to increase control over the conditions and events that affect their health (World Health Organization, 1986). It is time to listen to the voice of the consumer. Lloyd and Beymer-Ludwig (1999) remind us that

> listening to the voice of the consumer provides clear messages about the expectations of those served. How providers respond to these data will set the tone for the future. Clients are the reason health care providers exist. (p. 109)

Summary

The general features of community primary health care delivery in the future will be (1) integrated systems that meet the needs of populations, not just patients; (2) an evidence-based approach that focuses on the entire continuum of care throughout the lifespan; and (3) public measurement and competition as an integrated system that incorporates the evaluation of service, access, and cost.

Integrated informational systems and care system processes will be designed to help clinical providers and community leaders with decision making focused on healthy people and building healthy communities. Partnerships that prioritize managing health risks in homes and neighborhoods together with empowering individuals and families to take responsibility for their own health will improve the health status of our populations and communities. Ultimately, local, regional, national, and global communities will be better served when we build an integrated delivery system centered around healthy people and healthy communities. Preventive services, holistic health practices, and collegial collaboration will be the priorities for the twenty-first century.

The best thing about the future is that it only comes one day at a time.
—Abraham Lincoln

REFERENCES

Bartlett, J. (1992). *Familiar quotations: A collection of passages, phrases, and proverbs.* Boston: Little & Brown.

Benson, H. (1979). *Timeless healing: The power and biology of belief.* New York: Scribner.

Benson, H. (1996). *The mind/body effect.* New York: Simon and Schuster.

Blumenthal, J. A., Jiang, W., Babyak, M. A., Krantz, D. S., Frid, D. J., Coleman, R. E., Waugh, R., Hanson, M., Appelbaum, M., O'Connor, C., Morris, J. J. (1997). Stress management and exercise training in cardiac patients with myocardial ischemia. Effects on prognosis and evaluation of mechanisms. *Archives of Internal Medicine. Vol 157* (19), 2213–2236.

Blyth, D. (1993). *Healthy communities, healthy youth.* Minneapolis, MN: Search Institute.

Davis, S. and Meyer, C. (1998). *Blur: The speed of change in the connected economy.* New York, NY: Warner Books.

Gordon, J. S. (1996). *Manifesto for a new medicine: Your guide to healing partnerships and the wise use of alternative therapies.* Reading, MA: Addison-Wesley.

Gordon, S. (1997). *Life support.* Boston: Little, Brown and Company.

Gottlieb, B. (Ed.). (1995). *New choices in natural healing.* Emmaus, PA: Rodale Press.

Hancock, T. & Garrett, M. (1995). Beyond medicine: Health challenges and strategies in the twenty-first century. *Futures, 27,* 935–951.

Heterick, R. C. (1997). Maybe Adam Smith had it right. *Academic Leader,* Vol. 13, No. 11 (November 1997), pp. 1–3.

Institute for Clinical Systems Integration. (1994). Pediatric and adult preventive services. Minneapolis, MN: Group Health, Inc.

Kreitzer, M. I. & Plotnikoff, G. (1997). Transforming health care: Integrating complementary, spiritual, and cross cultural care. Minneapolis: University of Minnesota.

Lewin, J. C. (1997). Setting the public health agenda for the twenty-first century. In *Conference proceedings: A barn raising for public health: Building on Iowa's heritage in the twenty-first century* (pp. 5–9). Des Moines: Iowa Department of Public Health.

Lloyd, R. & Beymer-Ludwig, P. (1999). Listening to faith communities: Collaboration with those served. In Solari-Twadell, P. A. & McDermott, M. A. (eds.). *Parish Nursing: Promoting whole person health within faith communities.* Thousand Oaks, CA: SAGE Publications.

Myss, C. (1996). *Anatomy of the spirit.* New York: Harmony Books.

Rogers, E. M. (1983). *Diffusion of innovations.* New York: The Free Press.

Satinsky, M. A. (1998). *The foundations of integrated care; Facing the challenges of change.* Chicago: American Hospital Publishing, Inc.

Senge, P., Kleiner, A., Roberts, C., Ross, R., Roth, G., Smith, B. (1999). *The dance of change: The challenges of sustaining momentum in learning organizations.* New York, NY: Doubleday Currency.

Westberg, G. (1990). *The three acts of illness* [Videotape]. Available from International Parish Nurse Resource Center, Park Ridge, IL.

World Health Organization. (1986). *The Ottawa charter for health promotion.* Copenhagen: WHO Regional Office for Europe.

APPENDIX A

Health Bond*

Appendix A includes an executive summary of information from **Health Bond: B**uilding **O**pportunities **N**ew **D**irections. The full report provides outcomes and lessons learned from a five-year grant for "Strengthening Hospital Nursing: A Program to Improve Patient Care." This project was supported in part by two of the nation's largest private foundations, The Robert Wood Johnson Foundation and the Pew Charitable Trusts.

Health Bond was a voluntary, noncontractual service and education partnership of three member hospitals—Immanuel St. Joseph's–Mayo Health System (formerly Immanuel–St. Joseph's Hospital) in Mankato, MN, the grantee; Arlington Municipal Hospital in Arlington, MN; and Waseca Area Medical Center (formerly Waseca Area Memorial Hospital) in Waseca, MN—and two partner higher education institutions, Minnesota State University, Mankato (formerly Mankato State University), Mankato, MN; and South Central Technical College, located in North Mankato, MN.

Health Bond formed a consortium that focused on **B**uilding **O**pportunities and **N**ew **D**irections for health care services in a nine-county rural region (see Figure A-1). Health Bond served as a catalyst for expanding patient care and family health beyond the walls of the hospital to meet the challenge of delivering accessible, quality health care and education cost-effectively.

The Health Bond consortium catalyzed action by participating organizations. A small staff worked with existing organizations facilitating education and collaboration at the organizational level and between organizations. The successes shared in the Health Bond story resulted from the efforts of many people in those organizations and the communities they served. These people were energized by a shared vision of meeting the health needs of individuals and families through a regionally integrated, quality, cost-effective health system. The Health Bond story will be useful to rural and urban health care providers who share responsibility for clients from rural areas along their life/health continuum.

Interactive planning, consumer focus, commitment to quality, cost-effective health care, and systems thinking all contribute to the outcomes described herein. Health Bond's shared vision of regional rural health has spread, using a shared decision-making structure to develop service and education partnerships and initiate organizational/interorganizational cultural change. Consultation, education, and training, made available to administrators, middle managers, and faculty, together with selected staff, contribute to culture change. Experiential learning programs focus on concepts and skills of communication, relationship management, leadership development, individual empowerment, primary care and collaborative decision making.

*For further information and complete document on **Health Bond,** contact the Office of Administration, Immanuel St. Joseph's–Mayo Health System, 1025 Marsh Street, P.O. Box 8673, Mankato, MN 56002-8673, Telephone (507) 345–2646, Fax (507) 345–2908,
Email: "Maczuga, Catherine" <maczuga.catherine@mayo.edu>

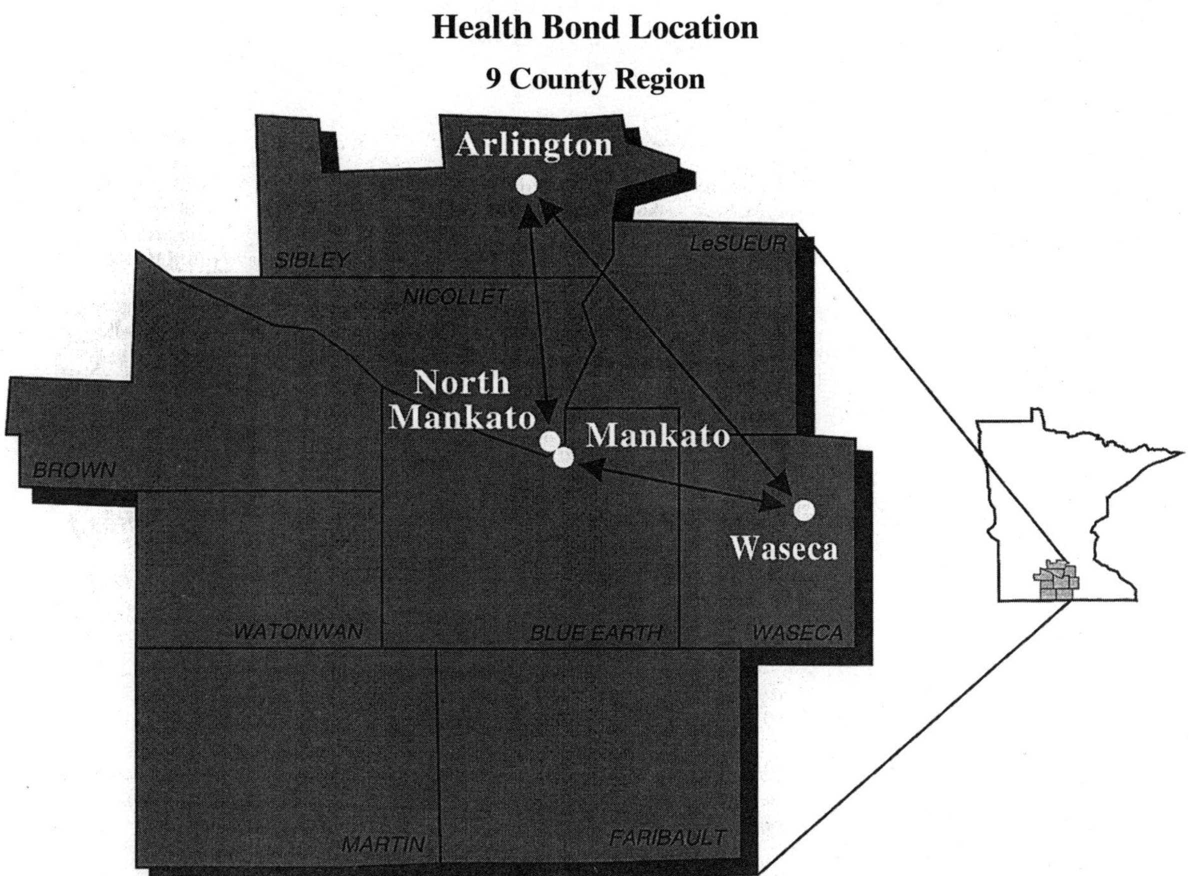

FIGURE A.1. Location of Health Bond Consortium Organizations. Boundaries of Region 9

Accomplishments resulting from collaborative work and the integrative nature of Health Bond's objectives include:

- Increased patient satisfaction, improved work environment, effectively managed costs
- Collaborative rural health professional educational programs
- Regional rural health cooperative in a nine-county South Central Minnesota region
- Community response-ability during life-threatening outbreaks of meningitis, legionnaires disease, and salmonella

Socio-political-economic change in society is swift and complex. Community integrated service networks are being implemented to assure accessible, quality, cost-effective health care responsive to the needs of rural and urban populations. Today's healthcare organizations seek to be proactive in creating integrated health care models for their community and region. Time is of the essence.

The Health Bond experience offers strategies which liberate the innovative ideas and leadership potential within individuals, work groups, and organizations. These strategies contribute to community network integration and regionalization of health care. We hope that these strategies applied, outcomes achieved to date, and lessons learned will assist you in the quest for your healthcare future. As one of Health Bond's Rural Primary Care Hospital nurse executives said, "The Journey is the Destination." The answers for you are within your own organization, community, and region.

The community and regional environment in which Health Bond organizations function are different from many others and different than just a few years ago. Changes in community and regional responsiveness and response-ability are much more than adding up many small changes, for the whole is greater than the sum of its parts. Developing community response-ability happens when:

- Opportunities are created for working together within/between agencies/organizations on shared goals, creating an atmosphere of trust and cooperation
- All parts of the community (individuals, families, groups, officials, agencies, organizations, populations) learn to work together in new and interdependent ways
- Trust grows through sustained mutual commitment to an end goal which is supported by each organization or agency
- Focus on the goal versus short-term interests creates community confidence and mutual support

Participants in the Health Bond Consortium created new environments of response-ability in our relationships with one another; within and between our organizations, providers, agencies in community, region. In the information age, traditional boundaries of agencies, organizations, and institutions are coming down. Each organization recognized the need to be involved in supporting the community and encouraging healthy lifestyles. No one organization is able to meet all of the needs. By working together, pooling knowledge/resources, those needs can be met as each participating organization becomes stronger as a result of the collaborative effort.

One of the first tasks of the Health Bond Partners was to develop a shared vision. This process resulted in the following vision for the region:

- Quality, cost-effective patient and family-centered care
- Integrated health care services
- Providers and employers of choice

Five objectives for attaining our vision were determined:

- Promote cultural change among members of the health care team to facilitate continuous quality improvement
- Integrate a regional network of service and education providers
- Develop indicators to measure improvement in the quality and cost-effectiveness of care and service throughout the redesign process
- Improve coordination of services to promote a continuum of patient and family-centered health care
- Provide leadership through an interactive planning process for developing a regional healthcare system responsive to rural customers

Consortium Name and Logo

The consortium name is significant. Consortium participants chose the name Health Bond because it conveys the consortium's commitment to working together to provide quality health care to the region. The letters of the word 'Bond' are an acronym for Health Bond's slogan—'**B**uilding **O**pportunities **N**ew **D**irections'. Operating under an interorganizational shared governance structure, Health Bond member institutions worked collaboratively to catalyze changes in area health care delivery and health care provider education systems. Health Bond created avenues for people who hadn't worked together before to gather at the same table, energizing grass roots leadership. The resulting changes reflect innovations in:

- Service/education partnership development
- Structures and strategies for creating change
- Designing services for a client focused continuum of care
- Regionalization of health care and education

The three sides of the logo represent the three founding hospitals and the interdependence they have created as a consortium. In addition, the three sides portray the three components central to Health Bond's mission—service, education, and partnership.

The story of the development of the name and logo for the consortium illustrates the teamwork and cooperation which emerged over the past six years. This spirit of cooperation and collaboration among providers and consumers in South Central Minnesota guided consortium initiatives.

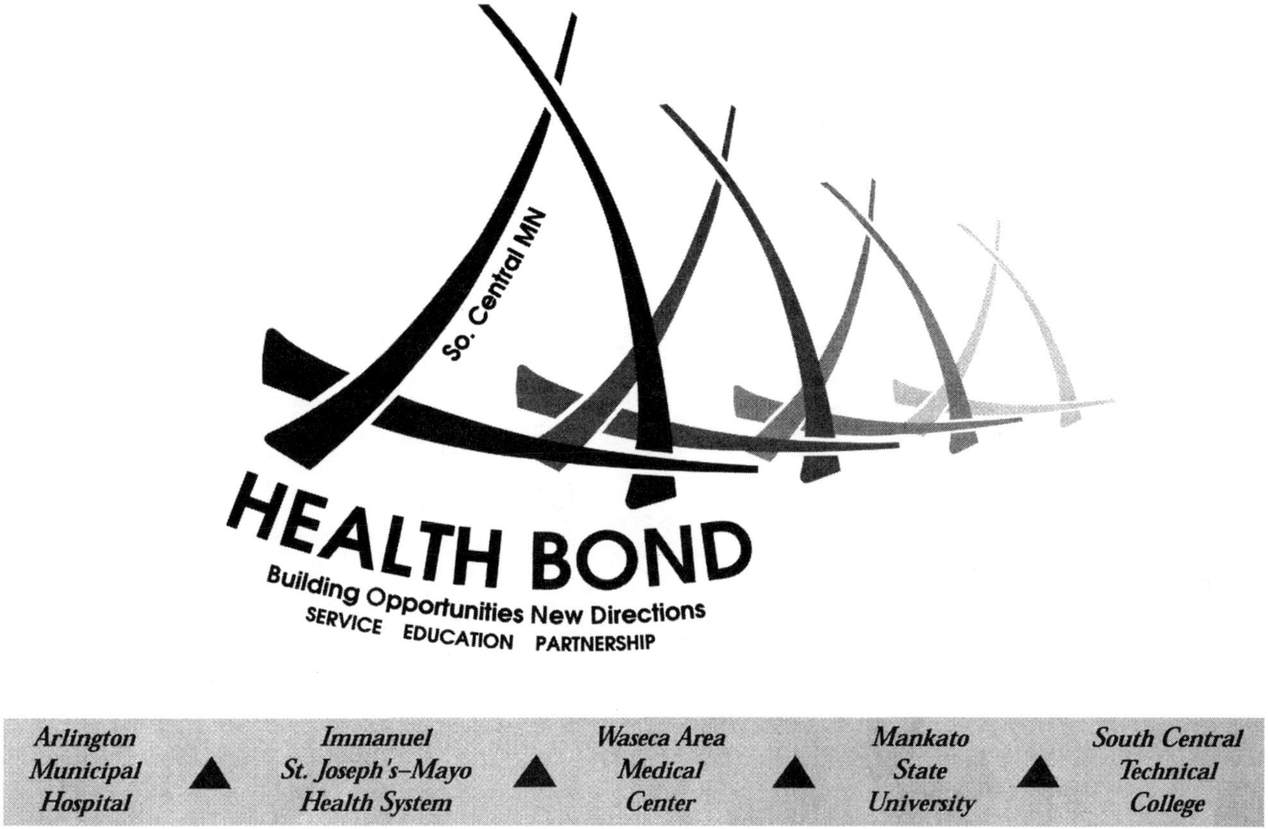

FIGURE A.2

From Aadalen SP, ed. Health BOND: Building Opportunities New Directions, Mankato, Minnesota, Health Bond, 1996. By permission.

APPENDIX B

Healthy People 2010*

Appendix B includes an executive summary of information from **Developing Objectives for Healthy People 2010,** a publication from the U.S. Department of Health and Human Services. An outline of the document is listed below:

- About This Guide
- What Is "Healthy People?"
- How Can Organizations and Individuals Contribute to Healthy People?
- What Is the Healthy Consortium and Who Are Its Members?
- Schedule of Healthy People 2010 Development
- How Should Healthy People 2010 Be Structured?
- Types of Objectives
- Criteria for Objectives Development
- Call for Comments
- The Secretary's Council on National Health Promotion and Disease Prevention Objectives for 2010
- The Healthy People Steering Committee
- Healthy People Work Group Coordinators
- Appendix A: Consortium Members
- Appendix B: Summary List of Year 2000 Objectives
- Appendix C: Resource Publications List

Healthy People 2010 Fact Sheet

All Americans have the opportunity to build the nation's health agenda for the 21st Century. Developing the objectives for Healthy People 2010 offers individuals, private and voluntary organizations, businesses, and the public health community the opportunity to help define the critical measures the United States must undertake to promote healthy behaviors, achieve improved health outcomes, reduce risk factors, and assure access to preventive strategies and health services that can improve the health of all Americans.

The first set of national health targets was published in 1979 in *Healthy People: The Surgeon General's Report on Health Promotion and Disease Prevention.* Healthy People 2000, the second and current national prevention initiative, is the product of unprecedented collaboration among government, voluntary and professional organizations, businesses, and individuals. Healthy People's national targets have served as the basis for monitoring and tracking

* For further information and complete document contact Department of Health and Human Services, Office of Disease Prevention and Health Promotion, Hubert H. Humphrey Building, Room 738G, 200 Independence Avenue, S.W., Washington, DC 20201, Telephone (202) 205–8583.

health status, health risks, and use of preventive services. Many states and localities have used the same process to guide local public health policy and program development.

Development of Healthy People 2010 has begun with members of the Healthy People Consortium, an alliance of over 600 national membership organizations representing professional, voluntary, and business sectors, and state and territorial public health, mental health, substance abuse, and environmental agencies. Overall development of Healthy People 2010 is guided by the Secretary's Council on Health Promotion and Disease Prevention Objectives for 2010. Chaired by the Secretary of HHS, with the Assistant Secretary for Health as Vice Chair and composed of former Assistant Secretaries for Health and all HHS Operating Division Heads, the Council meets annually.

Healthy People Homepage: More information about Healthy People 2010 developments and Healthy People 2000 activities is posted on the Internet at **http://odphp.osophs.dhhs.gov/pubs/hp2000.** Also at this website is the guide *Developing Objectives for Healthy People 2010,* which describes the who, what, when, and how of the 2010 development process. Included in this publication are the names of people in Federal and State agencies who coordinate Healthy People activities, as well as contact information for organizations that are members of the Healthy People Consortium.

Development of Objectives: There were two separate public comment periods on Healthy People 2010. In the fall of 1997, a call for comments on the proposed framework of Healthy People 2010 was announced in the *Federal Register,* as well as a call for objectives. Individuals were able to submit comments on current Healthy People objectives—proposing modifications and/or deletions—or submit new draft objectives before December 15, 1997. Comments were accepted electronically at: **http://web.health.gov/healthypeople.** Once the comment period closed, HHS work groups developed the 2010 draft.

A second public comment period on the draft Healthy People 2010 document was scheduled for the fall of 1998. Publication of *Healthy People 2010* is slated for early 2000.

For more information about Healthy People 2010, contact the Office of Disease Prevention and Health Promotion, Room 738G, Hubert Humphrey Building, 200 Independence Avenue, S.W., Washington, DC 20201 at (202) 205-8583.

About This Guide

You are invited to participate in the process of developing Healthy People 2010, the third set of national health promotion and disease prevention objectives. This guide includes background on the Healthy People initiative, who is involved, a calendar of major events, and ways the public can help develop objectives.

This guide is a resource for individuals and groups to use in reviewing and modifying year 2000 objectives, as well as developing new objectives. Proposed objectives and comments on the proposed structure were submitted through December 15, 1997. In the fall of 1998, a draft of Healthy People 2010 objectives was circulated for public review and comment. We encouraged everyone to participate in these and other Healthy People 2010 development activities to ensure that this initiative reflects the broad scope of public health in the United States.

This guide is intended for use by private and voluntary organizations; local and state public health, mental health, substance abuse, and environmental agencies; Federal government agencies; and any individual interested in improving public health. Because Healthy People is national in scope, everyone is encouraged to participate in developing the objectives that will guide prevention efforts into the next millennium.

What Is "Healthy People"?

For two decades, the U.S. Public Health Service (PHS) has used health promotion and disease prevention objectives to improve the health of the American people. The first set of national health targets was published in 1979 in *Healthy People: The Surgeon General's Report on Health Promotion and Disease Prevention.* This set of five challenging goals, to reduce mortality among four different age groups—infants, children, adolescents and young adults, and adults—and increase independence among older adults, was supported by objectives with 1990 targets that were designed to drive action. Through the combined efforts of the Nation's public health agencies, the 1990 targets set for infants, children, and adults were achieved. Adolescent mortality did not decline sufficiently to reach the 1990 target, and data systems could not adequately track the older adults' target.

Healthy People 2000

Healthy People 2000 built upon the lessons of the first Surgeon General's report and is the product of unprecedented collaboration among government, voluntary, and professional organizations, businesses, and individuals. Several themes distinguished Healthy People 2000 from past efforts, reflecting the progress and experience of 10 years, as well as an expanded science base for developing health promotion and disease prevention objectives. Many of the year 2000 objectives specify improving the health of groups of people bearing a disproportionate burden of poor health compared to the total population.

The framework of Healthy People 2000 consists of three broad goals:

1. Increase the span of healthy life for Americans
2. Reduce health disparities among Americans
3. Achieve access to preventive services for all Americans

Organized under the broad approaches of health promotion, health protection, and preventive services, the more than 300 national objectives are organized into 22 priority areas. This framework provides direction for individuals to change personal behaviors and for organizations and communities to support good health through health promotion policies. This framework can be envisioned as a house with a foundation of surveillance and data systems, rooms with Healthy People 2000 priority areas, and a roof that encompasses the three goals (see Figure B-1).

Year 2010 Objectives

The context in which Healthy People 2010 is being developed differs from that in which Healthy People 2000 was framed—and will continue to evolve throughout the decade. Advances in preventive therapies, vaccines and pharmaceuticals, assistive technologies, and computerized systems will all change the face of medicine and how it is practiced. New relationships will be defined between public health departments and health care delivery organizations. Meanwhile, demographic changes in the United States—reflecting an older and

Note: See Fig. 2.1 Vision of 2010: Healthy People in Healthy Communities, Chapter 2, Models for Building Healthy Communities.

HEALTHY PEOPLE 2000 GOALS

- Increase the span of healthy life for Americans.
- Reduce health disparities among Americans.
- Achieve access to preventive services for all Americans.

HEALTHY PEOPLE 2000 PRIORITY AREAS

Health Promotion

1. Physical Activity and Fitness
2. Nutrition
3. Tobacco
4. Substance Abuse: Alcohol and Other Drugs
5. Family Planning
6. Mental Health and Mental Disorders
7. Violent and Abusive Behavior
8. Educational and Community-Based Programs

Health Protection

9. Unintentional Injuries
10. Occupational Safety and Health
11. Environmental Health
12. Food and Drug Safety
13. Oral Health

Preventive Services

14. Maternal and Infant Health
15. Heart Disease and Stroke
16. Cancer
17. Diabetes and Chronic Disabling Conditions
18. HIV Infection
19. Sexually Transmitted Diseases
20. Immunization and Infectious Diseases
21. Clinical Preventive Services

22. Surveillance and Data Systems

FIGURE B-1 Healthy People 2000 Framework

more racially diverse population—will create new demands on public health and the overall health care system. Global forces—including food supplies, emerging infectious diseases, and environmental interdependence—will present new public health challenges.

Development of the year 2010 objectives has already begun with the users of the current objectives. At the November 1996 meeting of the Healthy People 2000 Consortium in New York City, the theme was "Building the Prevention Agenda for 2010: Lessons Learned." This meeting was complemented by focus group sessions where Consortium members discussed the current framework, goals, and objectives to assess the improvements needed to make the

2010 agenda relevant to the first decade of the 21st century. A report on the focus group findings can be found on the Healthy People 2000 Homepage at **http://odphp.osophs.dhhs.gov/pubs/hp2000.**

This next set of national objectives will be distinguished from Healthy People 2000 by the broadened prevention science base; improved surveillance and data systems; a heightened awareness and demand for preventive health services and quality health care; and changes in demographics, science, technology, and disease spread that will affect the public's health into the 21st century. The widespread use of the year 2000 objectives by states, localities, and the private sector also provides a base of experience upon which to build. While the Federal Government will take the lead in developing the initial draft objectives, this process is designed to be very participatory.

Healthy People 2010 is the United States' contribution to the World Health Organization's (WHO) "Health for All" strategy. The U.S. effort will be characterized by intersectoral collaboration and community participation. Through national objectives, the United States can provide models for world policy and strategies for population health improvement.

APPENDIX C

Los Angeles Times Articles

Note: Columns continue on next page. Read top to bottom across two pages throughout Appendix C.

SUNDAY, MAY 7, 1995, PART A, PAGE 1

COLUMN ONE

Outbreak Strikes a Small Town

■ **The first two cases of meningitis might be coincidental, Mike Osterholm thought. But the third sent Minnesota's top disease sleuth to Mankato to battle a familiar—and deadly—foe.**

By BARRY SIEGEL
TIMES STAFF WRITER

MANKATO, Minn.—The phone call Mike Osterholm received early Saturday morning, Jan. 28, was not for him all that unusual. It looks like we have two cases of bacterial meningitis, a state disease surveillance specialist was saying. Two sick teen-agers, down in Mankato, the seat of Blue Earth County.

written about it, he'd studied it, he'd fought it. He knew how it behaved. He thought of it as an old, familiar relative.

But the familiar relative had been acting strangely of late.

For reasons unknown, Group C outbreaks had risen sharply since 1991. On Osterholm's desk that weekend, newly arrived, sat the Feb. 1 edition of the Journal of the American Medical Assn. In it, an article described 10 such outbreaks in the United States in the past 2 1/2 years. There had been only six in the eight years before that. The rate had quadrupled.

"An emerging threat. . .," JAMA called these outbreaks. "One of the most feared public health emergencies, in part because of the disease's ability to strike, seemingly at random, previously healthy persons, killing one of every seven affected."

Meningococcal disease, Osterholm knew, was one of the few that could take cases involved the same bug—Group C *Neisseria meningitidis.*

Dammit, Osterholm thought. Here we go. We've definitely got something now.

What he had, in fact, was an outbreak unprecedented in all the scientific literature. Before it ended six weeks later, the *Neisseria meningitidis* bacteria would behave in Mankato in ways never before reported. In turn, the Minnesota Health Department and the Mankato community would wage a battle never before attempted. There would be moments of panic, accomplishment and tragedy. Most of all, there would be uncertainty. When the bacteria's siege finally abated in mid-March, it would remain unclear just who had won.

Armed with state-of-the-art tools, guided by years of experience, the experts could study, poke and assault the bug, but they could not explain or master it. Forced to navigate uncharted waters,

As Minnesota's state epidemiologist, Osterholm hears such reports fairly often. Most don't amount to anything but isolated illness.

Osterholm was about to leave his Minneapolis home to run errands. It was Super Bowl weekend. Divorced, he had his two children over. He planned to watch the game with his 13-year-old son, Ryan.

They don't even know if these two cases are related, Osterholm told himself. They don't even know if it's the same bug.

Still, he hesitated.

At 42, Osterholm had been Minnesota's top medical sleuth for 11 years. He'd developed a national reputation as one of the country's premier experts in tracking and controlling infectious disease. "If anyone is going to pay me a compliment when I die," he liked to say, "I hope it's that I learned to think like the bugs do."

Osterholm believed he understood the bug—Group C *Neisseria meningitidis*—that caused most outbreaks of meningococcal disease. He'd

Outbreak Strikes a Small Town. FIRST OF TWO PARTS

a healthy person and, by infecting the bloodstream or the lining around the brain and spinal cord, kill within six hours. You could go to bed with flu-like symptoms and never wake up.

Osterholm didn't want to over-respond to the news from Mankato, didn't want to foment panic. He also, though, didn't want to underestimate the problem.

Let's get blood samples up to the state lab, he told his staff that Saturday. Let's get more clinical information about the patients. Let's set up a conference call. Let's contact the schools down there.

Then he waited for his old familiar relative to show its hand.

The wait lasted just one night. On Sunday morning, Osterholm's phone rang again. The Mankato hospital now had a third case of meningitis. And the state lab now had a result: The first two

they could not know whether they were choosing the right course. In the end, they could not even say for sure whether they'd had any impact at all.

Of only one issue was Osterholm utterly certain: "Mankato is not the exception," he declared. "It will be the norm."

The Basketball Player

When Joe Kratzke arrived home at 10 p.m. on Thursday, Jan. 26, he told his father he felt "kind of achy" and wanted to stay home from school part of the next day. Kratzke, 17, a lanky 6-foot-2 and 175 pounds, was the shooting guard on Mankato West High's basketball team. They had a game Friday night. He wanted to be rested.

His father, Gary, was irritated. If Joe didn't feel well, why had he stayed out so late?

It was a challenge for Gary. At 45, he had to run the family's retail clothing store while rearing three children. His wife, Julie, had died of cancer almost exactly a year before. Besides Joe there was Jill, 11, and Justin, 9.

OK, he told his son. But you've got

to spend part of the day at school or they won't let you play.

The next day, Joe went to school from noon to 3 p.m. When his father came home at 5:30, he found Joe sleeping. He woke him and gave him a bowl of soup. Joe was sluggish. He had a headache.

Mankato West requires its varsity players to be at the gym in time to watch the B game, so Joe drove to the school at 6. Gary followed soon after. Sitting in the stands looking at his son as he walked by, he noticed that Joe had rashes on the inside of both arms.

In warm-ups, Joe appeared lethargic. He, Gary and the coach conferred. How do you feel? Gary inquired.

By then, Joe's head was exploding with pain every time he ran, every time his foot hit the ground. His neck felt sore, his legs stiff and tired. He knew he couldn't play, but didn't want to say so. Finally, he had to. "Well, this headache is pretty bad," he allowed.

As Joe sat on the bench watching the game, the rash on his arms began spreading. He grew faint, and pale and scared. At halftime, he decided he wanted to see a doctor right away.

serious. But Joe's rash troubled Nolan. It was the kind they saw in meningitis.

Large Group C epidemics occurred in the United States up until 1944; an estimated 2,600 cases and more than 370 deaths still occur each year. Most arise in the fall and winter; most affect school-age children and young adults, probably because their immune systems are still developing.

Until a few years ago in Mankato—a small river town of 31,000 about 80 miles south of the Twin Cities—doctors used to see 10 or more meningitis cases a year. Then, in the mid-1980s, they started giving infants a new vaccine for Type B influenza, which involves a similar bug. Ever since, they hadn't seen much meningitis at all.

But tonight they were, Nolan surmised. Fever, vomiting, headache, stiff neck, confusion, sleepiness, irritability and rash—these were the classic symptoms.

Admitting Joe to the critical care unit, the doctor ordered massive doses of penicillin and a second antibiotic. He knew, however, that the medicine might not save Joe. Even if it killed the bacteria, the dying bugs would keep produc-

The Bandleader

It was not until early Saturday that the hospital staff realized they might have two meningitis cases on their hands.

Sara Kleinsasser, a 17-year-old Mankato West High bandleader, had arrived at Immanuel-St. Joseph's more than two hours before Kratzke. When admitted at 6:13 p.m. she'd been feverish, limp, delirious and covered by a bruise-like rash. Doctors had labored for hours to stabilize her plummeting blood pressure, but had not fixed on a definite diagnosis.

Reporting for duty at 7 on Saturday morning, bedside nurse Maurine Corcoran and nursing supervisor Mary Guentzel heard about both Joe and Sara.

They decided they should call Jane Schwickert, the hospital's infection control nurse practitioner. By 9:15 a.m., Schwickert was at the hospital, peering over Sara and Joe. Both were in respirator isolation, both were comatose. Sara's blood pressure was dropping fast.

If this was the start of an outbreak, how to control it? Should they give antibiotics to all close contacts of these patients? Which one? What was the proto-

Accompanied by his girlfriend, Joe left the game at 8:30 and drove to nearby Immanuel-St. Joseph's Hospital. Walking the last 100 feet across the parking lot to the outpatient lobby, he vomited six times.

At a glance, nurse Kelly Duncanson knew to get Joe to the emergency room. There, because of the severe headache, Dr. Andy Boggust ordered a CAT scan, which revealed nothing unusual. The ER doctor considered: Joe's temperature was rising. The rash indicated bleeding under the skin. It looked as if they were dealing with an infectious process.

Boggust ordered a spinal tap. That revealed cloudy spinal fluid—it normally is clear—and spinal fluid pressure off the scale. This, the doctor now knew, was a disease process affecting the brain lining.

By then, Joe had started sinking into a dulled, semiconscious state. Dr. Peter Nolan, the emergency room's on-call pediatrician, had to rake his knuckles hard across Joe's chest to get any response.

Joe's cloudy spinal fluid could mean various types of infection, not all terribly ing deadly toxins.

Nolan took some comfort from Joe's elevated white-cell count. Good, he thought. That means he still has soldiers fighting for him.

Called by Joe's girlfriend, Gary Kratzke rushed to the hospital, where he found his son barely conscious. To him, Joe looked like a vegetable.

For nearly half an hour, the father talked to the son, sometimes eliciting brief responses. Then Joe started declining before Gary's eyes. Asked by a nurse, he could not speak his last name. Within minutes, Joe was in a coma. When Nolan knuckled him in the chest, he didn't respond at all.

Gary felt himself unraveling. I can't believe this is happening, he thought. I was just talking to him.

Shortly after midnight, Nolan took Gary aside. "This is a very frightening case," the doctor advised. "This is life or death. Joe could die."

At 2:30 a.m., just before leaving for home and his two younger children, Gary studied his son. Joe, he observed, looked just like his wife did when she passed away.

col?

Uncertain, feeling panicky, Schwickert decided to phone the state Health Department in the Twin Cities. Within two hours she was on a conference call, talking to Osterholm.

Schwickert felt impressed and reassured. Osterholm had a lustrous national reputation. He sat on countless committees and review boards, he projected unflappable assurance, he'd even tried twice—vainly—to swim the English channel. Reared in Iowa by an Irish mother and a Swedish father, he'd gone straight from college to the state Health Department, working there while he earned a master's degree in environmental health and a doctorate in epidemiology. He'd been tracking, writing and lecturing about bugs for 20 years.

On the phone, Osterholm led Schwickert and other Mankato officials through all the possibilities. Epidemiology 101, he called it. Much came from medical journal articles he'd coauthored.

Timing was important, he explained, in controlling both the outbreak and community panic. People should be careful, but not frightened. The bug spreads not through the air but through secretions of the nose and throat. So avoid deep kissing, don't share food or beverages, don't spray others with droplets from coughs or sneezes. But you can go to large gatherings such as sporting events.

They didn't know if it was really the same bacteria yet, Osterholm pointed out. They'd have to wait and see what developed. If they had a third case, the state would come down. Meanwhile, he wanted blood samples sent overnight to the Health Department's lab in Minneapolis for analysis.

For a time the next morning—Super Bowl Sunday—it looked as if Mankato might not be facing an outbreak after all. Joe and Sara still lay in the hospital's critical care unit battling for their lives, but they'd started to stabilize, and no new cases had arrived. After checking with the hospital, Schwickert went to brunch. Alice Weydt, the hospital's director of patient care, went to church. Osterholm's thoughts turned to the Super Bowl.

Then, close to 11:30 a.m., an ambulance rolled up to the emergency room door. Inside, flailing, throwing his arms

By midday, Osterholm was consulting with other state health officers who would be fighting the outbreak with him—among them Mike Moen, Kris Macdonald, Mary Sheehan, Craig Hedberg and Aggie Leitheiser.

By late afternoon, Osterholm was driving to Mankato.

He didn't know of any outbreak in which public health officials had started as quickly as they were. They had, he thought, a real chance of affecting the outcome in ways not normally seen. This is going to work, he told himself. This we're going to handle.

Then, driving on, he reconsidered.

Their foe was silent, cunning and invisible. Their foe was agent for the most formidable power of all—Mother Nature. Whatever they did, Osterholm had to admit, people were going to get sick, even end up blind or brain-damaged. Whatever they did, one in seven of their patients would likely die.

Battle Plan

We live in an age that promises an illusory safety, Osterholm likes to point out.

Most people grew up without much fear of or exposure to infectious diseases. Polio, tuberculosis, scarlet fev- health infrastructure, because of chronic underfunding and complacency in the age of antibiotics.

Driving to Mankato, reflecting on this situation, Osterholm seethed with frustration.

Microbes were sitting in the Twin Cities International Airport terminal that dwelt in African forests two days before. Almost 80% of the produce consumed in the United States was coming from developing nations. Minnesota, the whole country, was being bombarded from the outside. But scientists lacked the funds even to study properly what was happening.

The country's budget for disease surveillance was $75 million, and most of that went to AIDS, TB and sexually transmitted diseases. They had maybe $20 million for everything else, and Congress was talking about cutting funding for the Centers for Disease Control and Prevention and its infectious disease program. When something big broke, there just was no infrastructure to respond. It was like trying to run Chicago's O'Hare Airport with tin cans and string.

What he could do with the movie "Outbreak's" $45-million budget, Os-

about, was Jon Boyer, 17, a Mankato West student.

He'd had a sore throat all Saturday afternoon during his work shift at Jake's Stadium Pizza, his parents reported. At 8 p.m., he'd gone to a friend's house, but shortly after, not feeling well, he'd come home and climbed into bed. By 10:30, he was vomiting and feverish. By 3 a.m., he was delirious. By morning, his neck was so stiff he couldn't touch his chin to his chest.

Boyer had the classic symptoms of meningitis.

By the time Osterholm heard the news, he'd already received a call from his state lab. The samples from Mankato had arrived. Both looked to be Group C, the type most often involved in outbreaks.

Well, Osterholm reasoned, at least there's something to do now. A relatively rare vaccine did exist for Group C. It was not recommended for routine, general use because it didn't work with infants under 2, and didn't work with all types of the bug. It would work in Mankato, though.

er, influenza epidemics—they're all far in the past. So the public generally assumes modern medicine has licked infectious microbes, at least those that aren't obscure, exotic refugees from distant rain forests. If you get sick, unless it's something like cancer, you go to a doctor, you take medicine, you get better.

That, Osterholm knows, just isn't so. The world as he sees it looks far more perilous, its human inhabitants far more vulnerable. Microbes are continually evolving, and continually trying to consume our bodies. Malaria, AIDS, TB, E. coli, hantavirus, the so-called "flesh-eating" Group A strep—to epidemiologists, facing them is like trying to stop a juggernaut. Or, rather, slow it: Each year, about 100,000 people in the United States die of bacteria-induced toxic shock.

The microbes aren't spreading by evolution alone. Poverty, population explosion, disrupted ecosystems, international commerce—they all play a role. So, too, Osterholm argues, do relaxed surveillance and a collapse of the public

terholm fumed. Instead of Dustin Hoffman racing about in a helicopter, he had a crew of public health staffers scrambling to locate enough syringes. Instead of blank studio checks, he had staffers buying medicine by writing personal checks and pleading for $20,000 purchase orders.

Osterholm pulled into Mankato in the late afternoon. He couldn't help but relax a little in such a friendly, unpretentious place. Set in a wooded valley where the Minnesota and Blue Earth rivers join, Mankato is both a college town, home to Mankato State University, among other schools, and a processing center for a grain and livestock region.

There was good news for Osterholm at Immanuel-St. Joseph's.

At 3 p.m. Sunday, Gary Kratzke, encouraged by the hospital staff, had started talking to Joe, trying to draw a response from his comatose son. "Joe, can you hear me?" he'd repeated, standing at his son's bedside. "Joe, say something."

"What do you want me to say?" Joe

had finally answered, rolling his eyes. Even the doctors and nurses had cheered.

He's coming out of it, the hospital staff told Osterholm. Sara also was improving.

A 6 p.m. meeting of Mankato officials, called by Osterholm, drew a standing-room crowd of 40 to Immanuel-St. Joseph's education room. All sorts were there—hospital staff, private practice doctors from the Mankato Clinic, local politicians, county health officers, Mankato School District officials.

Osterholm flourishes before such gatherings; he is a polished public speaker. Educating and mobilizing communities is as central to his job as is studying bugs in the lab. It is also as tricky.

Osterholm stood before the Mankato crowd as an outsider, as an agent of the state. He was talking to medical doctors not inclined to take instruction from a Ph.D. So rather than direct, he guided toward consensus. Here's the situation, here are the options, here's what we know and don't know, he said. We're here to help. What do you want to do?

It worked. Those listening were impressed by his matter-of-fact knowledge community should be targeted for the vaccine? Since the disease usually affected youngsters who hung out together in places such as schools, should everyone from kindergarten through Mankato State University get vaccinated? Or just the district's junior and senior high students? Or only Mankato West students?

Should the antibiotic rifampin also be given? It sometimes was in meningitis cases, but its efficacy was uncertain, and it had various side effects. What's more, the antibiotic didn't protect you; rather, it reduced the chance of transmission. How to decide, when there was no broadly based study to show it made a difference at all?

Financial considerations couldn't be ignored—each vaccine costs $22. But the need to define and limit the response rose from more than just monetary issues. If they aimed too broadly, they'd be wasting time and diverting resources from the high-risk groups that most needed help. It would take a week or more to arrange 30,000 vaccines. Doing so, Osterholm felt, would be plain unethical. They couldn't delay getting the vaccine to those at highest risk. It was a triage issue; you treated those most in need first.

They would not, however, be given rifampin.

Osterholm marveled at this small town's mutual trust, enterprise, sense of community. Even as the meeting ended at 9:30 Sunday night, the hospital staff was scrambling to set up a hot line to handle calls from the community. School administrators were laying plans to distribute parent permission slips. Community relations specialists were herding reporters into a news conference. And Osterholm was on the phone to Connaught Laboratories in Swiftwater, Pa., ordering 4,000 doses of the Group C vaccine to be airlifted for Monday delivery.

The next 48 hours passed in a blur.

By 7 on Monday morning, Immanuel-St. Joseph's had a fourth meningitis patient—Casey Houston, a 16-year-old West High wrestler, whose parents thought he had the flu until, at 6:30 a.m., they read about the outbreak and discovered their son's neck was so stiff he couldn't bend it. By midmorning the hospital had a fifth case—an unidentified 64-year-old woman who'd been admitted on Saturday, but hadn't been diagnosed until now.

By midday, the media satellite

and appreciated the fact that he wasn't imposing his will. Perfect, thought Al Neely, the nurse manager of emergency and outpatient services. Super-impressive, thought Jerry Crest, the hospital's administrator.

Rather than inspire confidence in science, Osterholm had inspired confidence in himself. Later, he'd insist this made him uncomfortable, but in truth, it was needed, if only to curb panic. The science, after all, was not nearly as sturdy as Osterholm's poised performance.

In the days to come, they would be making decisions amid much uncertainty. They would have to move without the necessary information, before they had test results. They would have to act without knowing whether it was the right course.

The epidemiological literature suggests "extraordinary public health intervention" in meningitis outbreaks, including early "intensive selective vaccination campaigns." But "selective" is the operative word.

What segments of the Mankato

Osterholm also feared the slippery slope. If they started vaccinating people without a clear scientific basis, it was fairly easy to ask, why limit it at all? Why not vaccinate all of Minnesota? Already, seeds of panic were growing in Mankato. The TV stations were saying you needed to check your children every hour at night, they could die if symptoms were ignored. But it was January in Minnesota; there were lots of kids out there with flu or strep throat.

We need a rational reason for picking who we're going to vaccinate, Osterholm told those gathered Sunday evening.

The trouble was, a rational reason required an understanding of what linked those who'd gotten sick. That still wasn't apparent. The victims weren't close friends, did not play on the same teams, did not sit in the same classrooms.

So Mankato officials and Osterholm's staff mapped a plan based on what they did know. All junior and senior high school students in the district would get vaccinated Tuesday morning.

trucks had rolled into town, along with the first panicky rumors. By afternoon, a half-dozen school districts had canceled sporting events with Mankato teams. By day's end, dozens of nervous Mankato citizens had crowded into the Immanuel-St. Joseph's waiting room with flu-like symptoms, and more than 1,000 had called the hospital hot line.

The outbreak is not likely to spread beyond Mankato West High, Osterholm reassured the 300 citizens who attended a Monday evening community meeting in the school's auditorium. He did not recommend restrictions on travel. The risk is relatively small. "The real danger is not meningitis, but meningitis phobia," he said.

The vaccinations began Tuesday at 8:15 a.m. in the Mankato West High gym, directed by Nancy Meyer and Mary Gleason of the Blue Earth County Health Department. Within 34 minutes, 60 county health workers had inoculated more than 1,000 students. Within six hours, traveling by bus from school to school, they'd immunized the entire target group of 3,300.

That evening, much of Mankato collectively sighed in relief.

They had acted; they had countered the attack. They'd apparently saved five people—all the patients were improving—and the bug had not struck again.

As Wednesday, then Thursday, passed with no new cases, the media trucks pulled away, the calls abated. Although they knew the vaccine wouldn't take effect for 10 days, even the medical professionals began to feel pleased.

Nurse practitioner Schwickert went skiing Thursday night. School Supt. David Dakken began a rough draft of a thank-you letter to the medical community. We've licked this, hospital chief Crest told himself. "We are very definitely encouraged," Osterholm informed the local newspaper on Thursday.

As a hospital meeting ended at 7:30 the next morning, Friday, Feb. 3, Crest turned to Schwickert.

"I feel real good," he said.

"We've taken care of all these, and haven't lost one," Schwickert agreed.

rash, did she realize he likely had meningitis, even though he had been vaccinated three days before.

By the time she got him to Immanuel-St. Joseph's shortly after 7 a.m., he was too weak to walk. She rolled him through the emergency room door in a wheelchair. Still conscious and coherent, John asked his mother to turn on a television. Neither mother nor son realized just how sick he was.

The medical staff understood, though. Nurse manager Al Neely, observing the grape-colored bruises covering John's face and chest, sensed this boy was in trouble. When the initial lab work came in, Neely knew it.

Right on a slide, on the lab smear, he could see the microorganisms in John's blood that you'd usually have to grow out in a culture. You usually saw that only at a post-mortem. You don't expect to see that in a person who's talking to you.

If there were so many microbes in his blood that they could be seen, Neely knew that John's body had to be teeming with poison. John was awake, John was still talking to the doctors. But he'd need

By then, John's father, Basil, a business professor who'd been up in the Twin Cities, had reached the hospital. Shortly before 9 a.m., John told his parents he couldn't breathe. Minutes later, the hospital staff announced a "code blue" and began resuscitation efforts.

Two doctors called out instructions to critical care nurses and a respiratory therapist. Anesthesiologists monitored the airway and pumped oxygen. Nurse manager Neely—thinking of his own 16-year-old boy, who plays football at Mankato West—administered chest compressions. The hospital's vice president, Annette McBeth, after looking at John, warned the chaplain to get ready.

Linda and Basil couldn't believe this was happening. John was sick, but dying? Why? How? John was such a hustler, John had so much heart and soul.

Twice, three times, the staff got John's heart beating. He had no blood pressure, though, so he couldn't get the oxygen needed to keep going. After working on him for more than two

At that moment, a nurse, interrupting, leaned across the table. "Have you heard?" she said. "They've just brought another kid into the ER."

The Hockey Player

John Janavaras, 15, a scrappy, undersized Mankato West High hockey player who'd hustled his way onto the varsity team, had skated strongly during practice the day before. He'd felt safe enough to share a pop bottle with a friend after practice, despite public warnings. He'd felt well enough at 5 p.m. to make weekend plans to attend a hockey game. He'd felt hungry enough to call his mom and ask about supper.

An hour later, though, he was home in bed with a 102-degree fever, complaining of body aches. Classic flu symptoms, thought his mother, Linda, a Mankato-area gift shop owner. His friend and teammates had the flu days before; now it was his turn. She called the coach to say John wouldn't be at practice the next day.

Throughout the night, the mother checked on her son. Several times, John woke up. At 3 a.m., Linda gave him medicine for his fever. Not until 6 a.m., when she found her son covered with a miracle to survive.

The *Neisseria meningitidis* bacteria can be found residing benignly in the nasal passages of 1% to 4% of the population. For reasons unknown, the bug sometimes turns deadly and travels from the nasal passages to the bloodstream. Usually the immune system manages to eradicate it from the blood. The bug then goes to the spinal fluid and inflames the linings of the brain and spinal cord, causing meningitis.

As terrifying as that is, it's better than if the bug stays in the blood. Meningococcal septicemia—a blood infection—is much harder for doctors to treat. Even if they can kill the millions of rapidly multiplying bacteria in the blood with massive doses of antibiotics, they can't stop the dying bacteria from releasing their toxin into the blood, where it is carried to cells, tissues and organs, eventually destroying the entire human system.

That's what was happening to John. The bug was in his blood, not his spinal fluid. His small vessels were leaking, his pressure was dropping, clots were forming. He was in shock, his organs unable to get enough oxygen.

hours, doctors declared John dead at 11:39 a.m. As the news spread, doctors, nurses and administrators wept along with the parents.

"I didn't have a clue," Linda told a reporter days later. "I never imagined he would die. . . . No one took this (outbreak) seriously until John died. But these bugs, they do kill. . . ."

The medical staff was no less startled. They'd heard Osterholm describe the probabilities, but such vulnerability hadn't fit with what they'd held as true about their world. After saving five patients, they thought they'd be ready for another. They thought they were aware, and prepared.

They were not, McBeth now realized with dismay. To see someone rapidly decline as John did, second by second—she couldn't believe their efforts weren't working. That they were going as fast as they could, but couldn't go fast enough—it shook her to the core. She couldn't avoid feeling that, somehow, they'd all failed.

Those outside the hospital were even more shocked. That doctors and hospitals cured you when you fell sick had always been an article of faith.

The afternoon of John's death, Mankato West High Principal John Barnett agonized over how to announce it to his student body. "If you need to cry, cry," he finally urged over the public address system minutes after the lunch hour. "If you need to be with somebody, come to the auditorium." Hundreds did just that, hugging, weeping, gathering in small groups.

"As lay people," school Supt. Dakken would later observe, "we still hadn't grasped the swiftness and seriousness of the disease. To me, with John's death, it now hit home. I realized, however good you are, whatever your resources, regardless of what you do, you can't avert tragedy. . . . I hadn't realized that."

Less than half an hour after John's death, calls started flooding the hot line. They would be dealing with community panic, deflated hospital staffers quickly realized, as well as a rampant bug. It was a whole new ballgame.

Just then, news reached them that minutes before John died, a very sick 3-year-old boy had arrived at the emergency room with all the symptoms of meningitis. To McBeth, it now felt as if hell was breaking out. To Schwickert, it felt as if the world was collapsing.

bacteria.

(BEGIN TEXT OF INFOBOX / INFOGRAPHIC)

Outbreak in Mankato

Here is the timeline of the first days of the outbreak of meningitis cases in Mankato, Minn., and the extraordinary efforts health authorities had to make to contain the disease.

FRIDAY, JAN. 27

6:13 p.m. Sara Kleinsasser, 17, is admitted to Immanuel-St. Joseph's Hospital with symptoms later diagnosed as meningitis. Two hours later, Joe Kratzke, 17, is hospitalized after feeling ill during basketball game.

SATURDAY, JAN. 28

6:50 a.m. Hospital lab identifies bacteria as *Neisseria meningitidis.* State Department of Health is notified later in the morning.

11:45 a.m. Unnamed 64-year-old Mankato woman is third person admitted with symptoms later diagnosed as meningitis.

SUNDAY, JAN. 29

11:42 a.m. John Boyer, 17, is admitted with meningitis symptoms.

6 to 9:30 p.m. State epidemiologist Michael Osterholm holds meeting with medical personnel and local officials at

11:30 a.m. A 3-year-old boy, related to a West High student, is admitted with symptoms related to the meningitis bacteria.

11:39 a.m. John Janavaras dies.

5:45 p.m. Health and school officials decide to distribute the antibiotic rifampin to West High students. The hot line gets 708 calls.

Source: Jane Schwickert, Immanuel-St. Joseph's Hospital, Mankato.

To Osterholm, though, it felt as if they were traveling on a well-mapped road. The 3-year-old was the seventh case. One in seven had died, just as he'd warned. His old familiar relative was operating precisely by the book.

NEXT: The bug jumps the fire line.

(BEGIN TEXT OF INFOBOX / INFOGRAPHIC)

Glossary of Terms

* Meningococcal disease: A variety of serious infections, including meningitis, bacteremia and a form of pneumonia.

* Meningitis: A type of meningococcal disease. It is an infection of the brain lining and covering of the spinal cord. It can be caused by various viruses and bacteria, among them *Neisseria meningitidis.*

* Group C neisseria: One of four groups of the bacteria, the one involved in most outbreaks.

* Bacteremia (or septicemia): Any infection of the blood.

* Meningococcemia (or meningococcal septicemia): Blood infection caused by the *Neisseria meningitidis* hospital to discuss the diease and map strategy. After the meeting, the hospital sets up a meningitis hot line, and Osterholm orders 4,000 doses of vaccines for Monday delivery.

MONDAY, JAN. 30

7:12 a.m. Casey Houston, 16, is fifth patient admitted with meningitis symptoms.

In the evening, officials hold meetings at Mankato West and East high schools to discuss the disease and vaccination. Meanwhile, 1,093 people call the hot line.

TUESDAY, JAN. 31

8:15 a.m. to 2 p.m. Vaccination of seventh- to 12-grade students begins at Mankato West. Nurses then are bused to other students to continue vaccinations. The hot line gets 525 calls.

WEDNESDAY, FEB. 1

Follow-up vaccinations continue. The hot line gets 150 calls.

FRIDAY, FEB. 3

7:16 a.m. John Janavaras, 15, is admitted to hospital. Diagnosis: meningococcemia, a blood disorder caused by the same bacteria that causes meningitis.

MONDAY, MAY 8, 1995, PART A, PAGE 1

COLUMN ONE

Battling to Control a Killer Bug

■ A little town thought it had contained a meningitis outbreak. And then the disease took a surprising turn, plunging officials into a dilemma over how far to push the fight without pandering to panic.

By BARRY SIEGEL
TIMES STAFF WRITER

MANKATO, Minn.—It is the medical sleuth's constant quandary: How to respond before you know what you're officials who gathered late Friday afternoon, Feb. 3.

They felt sure that shutting down the school would be wrong. The bug wasn't being transmitted through the building, but through close social contact; the students would simply congregate off campus.

About the antibiotic, they were less sure. They didn't know if rifampin would do any good. It didn't protect those who took it, but rather, reduced the chance of transmission. It had never been used to combat an outbreak like this. And in the strong doses needed, it couldn't be given to people for extended periods.

For these reasons, Osterholm had resisted distributing the antibiotic earlier, hoping they'd quickly find and eliminate the source of the outbreak. They almost always did.

Mankato West's auditorium on Saturday, Feb. 4, the day after Janavaras died, 1,500 citizens—some plainly scared or irate—filled the main floor, balcony and aisles. A half-dozen parents accused officials of playing "Russian roulette" with their children's lives. Why hadn't they closed the school? they demanded. Why hadn't they vaccinated everyone? Why hadn't they given antibiotics from the start?

Osterholm's efforts to explain "a rational scientific basis" and "slippery slope" did not mollify everyone. On the phone that weekend, several callers threatened him, held him responsible, called him arrogant and uncaring. A Minneapolis TV station charged that Osterholm was losing Mankato's trust by giving the town "mixed messages" about risk and proper responses.

There were, in truth, only a handful

fighting? Timing is all. If everyone could breathe into the phone and provide instant lab results, Minnesota state epidemiologist Mike Osterholm likes to say, he could make incredible decisions. The trouble was, he had to act based more on the past than the present.

What to do now in Mankato?

Over one week in late January and early February, this small river town south of the Twin Cities had seven cases of deadly meningococcal disease and one death, a 15-year-old named John Janavaras. Despite a rapid response, despite giving 3,300 vaccinations to all junior and senior high students, officials had a classic outbreak on their hands.

Should they now expand the circle of who gets vaccinated? Should they start giving everyone the antibiotic rifampin? Should they close Mankato West High, where most of the stricken attend class?

Would doing so take them down a slippery slope? Or was it an aggressive but logical counterattack? Would they be caving in, pandering to community panic? Or would they be saving lives?

These were the type of questions facing Osterholm, his state Health Department colleagues and the Mankato

Not this time, though. Despite hours of interviews and detective work, they'd

Outbreak Strikes a Small Town. SECOND OF TWO PARTS

been unable to trace its genesis or figure out the links among the victims.

Experience indicated this outbreak would end without further action, Osterholm knew. But was that a reliable indicator?

In the end, Mankato and state health officials decided they just could not stand by idly. To buy time until the vaccines took effect in four days, they decided to give all junior and senior high students the antibiotic the next morning. What's more, on Monday they'd give antibiotics and vaccinations to 5,000 more people: Mankato West High's staff, the immediate family members of its students and staff, and those in close contact with its students.

Osterholm told reporters this response was "aggressive and unprecedented. . . . We're in uncharted waters." Not everyone applauded, however.

At a community meeting in

of critics speaking out, but they were having an impact. By now, Osterholm, much to his regret, was devoting half his time to putting out fires. Rumors were sweeping through Mankato.

Despite reassurances, two-thirds of Mankato West's students stayed away the Monday after Janavaras' death. (Not all remained at home, though; many gathered at the shopping mall or at friends' homes, just as Osterholm had feared.) Callers to the hospital hot line demanded the vaccine at whatever the cost. Callers to the Blue Earth County Health Department insisted that the vaccine itself was spreading the disease. Jake's Stadium Pizza owner Vernon (Sarge) Carstensen found it necessary to call a news conference to deny a widespread rumor that his wife, Norma, was the unnamed 64-year-old woman who was among the seven who had been hospitalized.

The agitation was even greater beyond Mankato's borders. Schools from across the state canceled sporting events. Shoppers packed the Wal-Mart in Blue Earth, 40 miles away, rather than visit Mankato's regional mall. Visitors canceled motel reservations. A store in

Wells, 34 miles to the south, refused a package delivered by a truck driver from Mankato.

A bus company wondered whether it should change its route through the area. An out-of-state candidate for a dean's position at Mankato State University canceled his scheduled interview.

A few treated Mankato West students—"Westies"—as lepers. A K mart shopper asked a checkout clerk where she went to school, then switched to another line when the answer was Mankato West High. One student wasn't allowed to come to work at the Civic Center for 10 days—until his vaccine became effective.

For a time, whenever the phone rang Mankato West Principal John Barnett flinched, fearing it was the hospital or Osterholm calling. Who's going to be next? Barnett wondered.

Then, once again, the furor abated. As the days passed without a new case, hot-line calls dwindled. When only 49 called on Friday, Feb. 10, a week after Janavaras' death, the hospital closed the hot line.

Osterholm now believed they were truly at the end of the siege.

didn't get any bigger," Osterholm said. "Just more and more lines connecting everyone in that group." Looking back, he told the reporters, the mass immunizations were probably "overvigorous," since the outbreak involved a small network from one school. But they hadn't known that, so their response was "prudent."

"I feel very confident today that we are out of the woods," Osterholm concluded. "This outbreak followed a road map exactly as we mapped it out. This thing had no real surprise punches."

The news that the outbreak had been traced to a small Mankato West group, the local Mankato Free Press editorialized two days later, "brings a sense of closure to a traumatic community event."

By the end of that week, Mankato West's attendance was back to normal and its athletic teams were back in action, no longer shunned by other schools. Osterholm was in Florida, vacationing with his children. You're done, he was telling himself. You're done.

He was not.

Move to New Level

After Jackie and Shayne Pitt's two Ryan had slept over at his house the night before. Ryan must have the flu.

At 7 a.m., Ryan fell into a more peaceful sleep and seemed better. So Jackie and her daughters left for church, leaving Shayne to care for his son.

At 11:30, Ryan woke and went into the bathroom. Shayne, looking in, saw 100 or more red pinpoint dots on Ryan's chest and the front of his legs. They resembled miniature chicken pox to Shayne, not the grape-colored bruises they'd been warned about.

Ryan had already had chicken pox, though.

Close to noon, Jackie returned from church. Come look at Ryan's rash, her husband said. Jackie looked, and froze. Let's get him to the hospital, she said.

As they were dressing Ryan, he started to mumble and say things that didn't make sense. The parents hurried. By the time Shayne was carrying Ryan to the car, the boy was delirious. His babbling grew ever stranger in the five minutes it took to get to Immanuel-St. Joseph's Hospital.

"He's acting like he has the flu, but he's got these dots on his body," Shayne started to tell the admitting nurse. The

They'd inoculated more than 5,000 at a second vaccine clinic the previous Monday. They'd discharged, over the course of the week, all the hospitalized patients: Joe Kratzke, 17; Casey Houston, 16; Sara Kleinsasser, 17; Jon Boyer, 17; a 3-year-old boy, and the 64-year-old woman. They'd finally linked the woman and the 3-year-old to Mankato West students, making their illnesses far less mysterious.

Osterholm felt certain they'd soon find the missing link among all those infected. "All these cases will tie together somehow," he told reporters.

At a news briefing the next Monday, he more or less announced that missing link, and declared the end of the outbreak.

They had found no smoking gun, he said. They couldn't trace the outbreak to a single person or event and didn't expect they ever would. But they had concluded that about 100 Mankato West students had played a role in the outbreak. They'd never met as a whole, but rather, had shared activities in varying alignments of five or six at a time.

"After the first 100, the diagram

teen-age daughters had been vaccinated in the first round of inoculations, Jackie had called the hospital hot line to ask if their 7-year-old son, Ryan, should also get the shot. No, she was told, not at this time.

That made sense to Jackie. This disease was hitting teen-agers, after all. And her daughters attended Mankato East High, not Mankato West.

Just 18 months before, the Pitts had moved to Mankato from Germany, where Shayne was a company commander in the U.S. Army. Now he taught ROTC at Mankato State. The family liked Mankato's small-town friendliness. Ryan, an exuberant second-grader at Kennedy Elementary School, had quickly learned to ice-skate and play hockey.

At hockey practice on Saturday, Feb. 26, he looked a little flat to his dad, but he played OK. Not until after he went to bed that night did he start to act sick. By the middle of the night, he was vomiting every half hour.

Jackie knew about the meningitis siege but wasn't too worried. The outbreak wasn't in Ryan's age group, she reasoned. His friend Jeff had the flu, and

nurse stopped writing. "I want the triage doctor to see him right away," she said.

In the emergency room, they gave Ryan steroids to reduce brain swelling, took blood samples, did a spinal tap. The on-call pediatrician, John Norris, ordered massive doses of penicillin. Then, as Ryan was being wheeled to the critical care unit, Norris approached Jackie and touched her on the arm.

"Are you OK?" he asked.

Six other cases ended up OK, Jackie was thinking. So yeah, she was OK.

Norris spoke gently. "This is the form of the disease where the bacteria is in the blood, not the brain," he said.

Jackie understood. She knew that was the form John Janavaras had.

"The first 72 hours will be critical," Norris said. "This is a matter of life and death. Ryan could die."

Jackie wept.

In critical care, Ryan's blood pressure was dropping as his body, in shock from the bacteria's toxin, bled internally. He wanted to nap, but the staff, fearing he'd stop breathing, kept talking to him. So did his mother. Ryan, garrulous as ever, responded.

He talked about a girl who hit him in the eye with a block at school. He ran through his Christmas wish list—Rollerblades, a pocketknife. He weighed possible birthday presents for his mom.

"Maybe I'll give you earrings," he told her. "Just like last year."

When they announced "code blue—CCU" on the loudspeakers shortly after 8 p.m., Jackie was down the hall, Shayne in a meeting room being interviewed by state public health officer Jan Forfang. "You better get in there," Forfang told Ryan's father.

Ryan had stopped breathing. A nurse, desperate, crying "We're losing him," had started mouth-to-mouth resuscitation, despite the danger to herself. A respiratory therapist had taken over a minute later with oxygen and fluids. By the time Shayne and then Jackie burst into the room, though, Ryan was breathing again. "Mom," he said, "it looks like you've been crying."

Norris ordered fresh frozen plasma and a medication to boost blood pressure. He also urged that Ryan stay awake. If the boy "coded" a second time, Norris would have to anesthetize him and put him on a respirator.

was easily the most unsettling and ominous of all they'd seen in Mankato. Until now, he'd felt sure they were traveling a familiar if dreadful road. Suddenly, the terrain looked strange.

Based on everything he knew, Osterholm had always assumed this bug would stay confined to linked individuals at a single institution—Mankato West High School. In the epidemiological literature, that's how it always worked. Ryan, though, had no apparent links to the other cases; he came from a different age group, a different social setting.

It looked as if this bug had now moved to a broader, more random population. An institutional outbreak had evolved into a community outbreak, which meant it might continue for many months. That had never happened before.

At meetings with Mankato officials, Osterholm found himself for once fueling rather than quelling concern. Well, you told us there'd be sporadic cases, some said. Osterholm had to be honest.

"I meant connected to Mankato West High," he said. "This has jumped the fire line. It's like it jumped to another forest."

demonstrated in the United States. . . . The outbreak has moved to a new level. . . . This type of shift has never been documented in any previous outbreak of meningococcal disease."

The public health team's determination to act only on a rational, scientific basis was eroding.

More than 1,000 calls a day once again flooded the hot line. Those from outsiders now included a few demands that they "close down" Mankato. Some used the word "quarantine." MSU students' parents questioned whether to let them come home. Truckers from Illinois refused to deliver ad inserts to the Mankato paper.

To those making decisions, the threat of mass hysteria seemed utterly real, and more than a little scary. The 18-year-old MSU student had been given penicillin before a blood sample was drawn, so they'd never really know if he had the outbreak bug. But they had to respond aggressively, they quickly decided—even if it was as much to quell community panic as to fight the bug.

They wouldn't just vaccinate the kids. Over four days, they'd vaccinate everyone 29 and younger in the Mankato

Do you have a girlfriend? asked the respiratory therapist posted at Ryan's bedside, struggling to keep the boy talking.

"Brittany," Ryan answered. "You know what I'm going to do when I see Brittany? I'm going to tell her I love her very much and she can do anything she wants to me."

Early in the morning, Ryan's blood pressure started to stabilize. Shayne noticed the room growing calmer. Staffers who'd stayed beyond their shifts started leaving. Soon Ryan was working his nurses, calling for root beer, hot chocolate and Froot Loops.

"I heard a nurse say, 'We're losing him,' " Ryan recalled. "I thought I might die, and my mom and dad would be crying." At 5 a.m., Jackie and Shayne settled onto cots and went to sleep.

By now accustomed to the recurring peril, the Mankato community at first responded calmly to the news of Ryan's illness. A town meeting in the Mankato West auditorium on Tuesday night, Feb. 28, two days after Ryan entered the hospital, drew a quiet crowd of 200.

To Osterholm, though, Ryan's case

The group quickly fixed on a plan. If genetic fingerprinting showed that Ryan's bug matched the strain in the other cases, they'd vaccinate all kids from preschool through sixth grade, about 4,500 total. While waiting for lab results, they'd get ready, make arrangements, reopen the hot line.

Late Wednesday, March 1, the state lab confirmed that Ryan's bug matched the others. Then, early the next morning, even more disturbing news arrived.

An 18-year-old Mankato State University freshman, Christopher Wilson, had been hospitalized in the Twin Cities with classic signs of meningitis. Wilson had no apparent link to Mankato West. He was from a Twin Cities suburb, he lived at MSU, he had no job in Mankato.

What in the world, Osterholm wondered, was going on?

He felt flat-out bewildered. He thought he knew this bug. He thought he could predict its behavior. It was like watching an old familiar relative act in an utterly bizarre way.

The bacteria's movement, he told reporters, "has never been previously

area—22,000 more in all. With that, they'd have inoculated half of the region.

Whether also to give everyone rifampin did draw some debate.

It wasn't just that rifampin had uncertain efficacy. It also had complications. It wasn't safe for pregnant women. It shouldn't be taken with alcohol. It negated birth-control pills. It sometimes caused side effects—diarrhea, headache, fatigue, vomiting, fever.

Still, they'd already given it to so many others in town. People would ask, why them, not us? People would demand it. People thought it protected them. It cost only 50 cents a dose.

They'd give rifampin to everyone, the Mankato and state health officials decided. They'd give it even if it was almost a placebo. They'd give it even though Osterholm's carefully constructed consensus was starting to weaken.

Among others, Jerry Crest, head of Immanuel-St. Joseph's, didn't think such a massive response was necessary medically. "Some of us frankly felt we shouldn't, that we didn't need to," he would later recall. "But we had to be consistent, we had to bring this to an end. There would have been such a reaction if we didn't. Parents of every college kid would be down here with guns. This was definitely an emotional reaction, based on mental health concerns."

Jane Schwickert, the hospital's infection control nurse practitioner, saw it a little differently. "It's not that we're going against science," she said. "It's that there isn't a whole lot of science there."

Osterholm saw it yet another way. True, they had no choice, the community required a response. "But the science was there," he insisted.

Late on Thursday, March 2, Jerry Crest appeared at the desk of Mary Bauer, in the hospital's material management department. "Mary," he began, "if I were to ask you for 20,000 syringes by tomorrow, can you do it?"

Laboring through the night, county and state health workers hand-counted antibiotic pills into 25,000 bottles. When the pediatrician who'd signed the order for the young children's medicine decided he was uncomfortable signing for adults, they had to find another doctor, then relabel every bottle with his name. When the new labels wouldn't stick, they had to start using Scotch tape.

seconds.

At 5 p.m. Monday, cheers and applause erupted as health workers administered the last of 23,452 vaccines. In all, public health officials had provided the vaccine and antibiotics to more than 30,000 since the outbreak began, at a cost of $1.03 million to the state and an equal amount to Immanuel-St. Joseph's and county health departments.

Still, not everyone was satisfied. Why not give vaccinations to the entire community? some demanded in phone calls and at a public meeting Monday on the MSU campus. Why not vaccinate people older than 29?

"I don't think you have to be Jonas Salk to figure this out," one MSU faculty member declared. "We're all at risk."

No, Osterholm flatly responded. He would not slip further down that slope; he would not divert resources from true health problems. Driving to the Twin Cities is riskier for adults than is meningitis.

Some nonetheless pressed: What about those willing to pay the entire cost themselves?

No, Osterholm said. They were done. They would conduct no more clinics.

Evolving Outlaw Bug

revelation this has been, people remarked, over and over. We didn't realize that this could happen.

Nothing Osterholm had to say could restore the town's lost sense of security. Instead, talking to about 40 medical and county officials gathered in Immanuel-St. Joseph's education room, he could offer only added mystery.

He didn't know why or how the outbreak had occurred, he allowed. He didn't know why some got sick while others didn't. He didn't know why one succumbed while others survived. Despite extensive follow-up, they'd never been able to link Ryan Pitt and the MSU student to the Mankato West cases. It was unlikely they ever would.

What they had learned, Osterholm revealed, was even more unsettling than what they had not.

During the last marathon vaccination round, they'd taken throat swabs from 3,000 elementary school children, seeking insights into the bug. Because this bacteria normally resides passively in the nasal passages of up to 4% of the population, in Mankato they'd expected to find it colonizing in hundreds of people, in order to get a few actual meningitis cases.

But out of 3,000 swabs, Osterholm

The next morning, the Red Cross brought coffee, food and water to the vaccination clinic at the Army Reserve Center in Mankato. The National Guard put up tents and directed traffic. The owner of A to Z Rental donated portable heaters. Grocery stores and restaurants donated food. Sixteen counties sent public health officials, 150 volunteers, scores of nurses. More than 3,000 citizens called the hot line, some asking for times and directions, others pleading.

Why not me, what about me? they implored. I'm two months past my 30th birthday. I work with kids.

By noon, 6,000 had converged in chill winter air at the Army Reserve Center, enduring traffic jams, shuttle buses and two-hour waits in a 400-yard-long line. On Saturday, with light snow falling and crying children huddling in parents' arms, officials increased the number of buses, expanded the vaccination stations from 14 to 25, added portable toilets, lights, tents. For 30 hours the marathon continued—781 shots per hour, 13 a minute, one every 2.2

Late in the day on March 16, Osterholm returned to Mankato to give a wrap-up summary of the outbreak, and what he called his "swan's song" to a community he'd come to admire greatly.

The town was more or less back to normal by then. There'd been no more cases reported, and the panic had abated. Joe Kratzke was playing basketball for Mankato West High, Ryan Pitt hockey for Kennedy Elementary. An early hint of spring had warmed the air, dispatching most sore throats and symptoms of flu.

Many talked about how proud and appreciative they were of their community for working together under such duress. Students wrote essays. Those who'd battled the bug planned a "post-meningital outbreak debriefing," with volleyball, boccie ball and music, at the Army Reserve Center, site of the last marathon vaccination session.

Lingering still, though, was a sense of vulnerability, a sense of a once-safe world now marked by constant, invisible, unavoidable peril. What a

reported, they had not found a single person carrying the outbreak bug.

The doctors listening in the education room exchanged glances.

That, they all knew, meant the bug was not running wild in the community. Rather, those few people the bug colonized, it made sick. This was, in other words, one extraordinarily virulent bug. This bug had an incredible ability to create severe disease.

Mankato had been hit not by a new bug, but an evolving bug—a representative of what the Journal of the American Medical Assn. editors and scientists were calling a "new clonal group in North America." It looked similar to a strain responsible for a doubling of meningitis cases in Oregon since 1991. Osterholm's old familiar relative was changing its personality.

Such evolution happens all the time, Osterholm knew, for a variety of reasons. Such is the world Darwin described. The more forcefully we attack the microbes, the more we accelerate the emergence of varied and resistant strains. We live in the bugs' world, they don't live in ours.

Yet something was strange in Mankato. It is not in a bug's best interest to kill off all its hosts, for it needs hosts. This one was doing just that, though. This one was an outlaw bacteria.

Bizarre, fascinating, scary—but it made sense. A new, more virulent outlaw bug would explain the dramatic increase in outbreaks in recent years. It would also explain why the Mankato outbreak had jumped its fire lines.

Of course, it would also mean that they most likely had not needed to spend more than $2 million and vaccinate 30,000 people, since the bug wasn't running rampant. They'd aimed far more broadly than the situation required.

If he had to do it over again, though, Osterholm told those gathered in the education room, he would do the same thing. Acting before information was available, what else could he do? "We had no choice," Osterholm said. "We didn't want to wait, then two weeks later find out this is what we should have done."

Left unsaid was another reason for the aggressive response. They acted as they did also because it was something they could do. The alternative—not to act—was simply unthinkable, both to health officials and the public.

was no time for further questions.

He was already late for another meeting, 80 miles to the east in Rochester. Another outbreak was under way there, this time of Group A strep—six cases, four deaths. Another town needed calming, another bug needed a response.

"We've forgotten the lessons of evolution," Osterholm said, juggling a beeper and cellular phone as he rushed through the hospital lobby toward his car. "The notion that we can dominate the world—Darwin never said that. It is misleading that we've had substantial gains against microbes in recent times. The truth is, it's not even halftime."

(BEGIN TEXT OF INFOBOX / INFOGRAPHIC)

Outbreak in Mankato

Here is the timeline of the outbreak of meningitis cases in Mankato, Minn., and the extraordinary efforts health authorities had to make to contain the disease:

FRIDAY, JAN. 27

6:13 p.m. Sara Kleinsasser, 17, is admitted to Immanuel-St. Joseph's Hospital with symptoms later diagnosed as meningitis. Two hours later, Joe Kratzke, 17, is hospitalized after feeling ill during a basketball game.

SATURDAY, JAN. 28

6:50 a.m. Hospital lab identifies bacteria as *Neisseria meningitidis.* State hospital's hot line.

TUESDAY, JAN. 31

8:15 a.m. to 2 p.m. Vaccination of seventh- to 12th-grade students begins at Mankato West. Nurses then are bused to other students to continue vaccinations.

The hot line gets 525 calls.

WEDNESDAY, FEB. 1

Follow-up vaccinations continue. The hot line gets 150 calls.

FRIDAY, FEB. 3

7:16 a.m. John Janavaras, 15, is admitted to hospital. Diagnosis: meningococcemia, a blood disorder caused by the same bacteria that causes meningitis.

11:30 a.m. A 3-year-old boy, related to a West High student, is admitted with symptoms related to the meningitis bacteria.

11:39 a.m. John Janavaras dies.

5:45 p.m. Health and school officials decide to distribute the antibiotic rifampin to West High students. The hot line gets 708 calls.

SATURDAY, FEB. 4

Joe Kratzke goes home from the hospital. Doses of rifampin are distributed to West Highstudents.

1 p.m.: Fifteen hundred Mankato citizens attend community meeting at Mankato West High auditorium to question Osterholm and others about the outbreak.

2:20 p.m.: Osterholm orders 5,500

Whether in fact they'd had any impact on the Mankato outbreak remains an unanswerable question.

It is "appropriate" to provide vaccines, a recent Journal of the American Medical Assn. editorial observed, but "unlikely to have substantial impact." Prevention will be an "elusive goal," the journal concluded, until an effective vaccine for routine use with infants is developed.

By starting early, Osterholm had hoped to alter this usual course of events. Had he?

Osterholm's best guess, based on previous outbreaks, is they prevented cases and deaths in Mankato. But it is hard, he allows, to say just what they did.

What about coming back to Mankato? asked one of the doctors at the meeting. What about swabbing more throats, doing follow-up studies, learning more?

No, Osterholm said, there was no time or resources for that. In fact, there

Department of Health is notified later in the morning.

11:45 a.m. Unnamed 64-year-old Mankato woman is third person admitted with symptoms later diagnosed as meningitis.

SUNDAY, JAN. 29

11:42 a.m. John Boyer, 17, is admitted with meningitis symptoms.

6 to 9:30 p.m. State epidemiologist Michael Osterholm holds meeting with medical personnel and local officials at the hospital to discuss the diease and map strategy. After the meeting, the hospital sets up a meningitis hot line, and Osterholm orders 4,000 doses of vaccines for Monday delivery.

MONDAY, JAN. 30

7:12 a.m. Casey Houston, 16, is fifth patient admitted with meningitis symptoms.

In the evening, officials hold meetings at Mankato West and East high schools to discuss the disease and vaccination. Meanwhile, 1,093 people call the more vaccine doses. The hot line gets 1,204 calls.

MONDAY, FEB. 6

Vaccinations and antibiotics are given to siblings and other family members of West High students during morning and afternoon shifts at Mankato East shopping center.

West High attendance drops to about a third of the 1,125 enrollment.

Casey Houston leaves the hospital.

The hot line gets 1,184 calls.

TUESDAY, FEB. 7

Sara Kleinsasser and John Boyer are discharged from the hospital.

The hot line gets 353 calls.

WEDNESDAY, FEB. 8

Funeral for John Janavaras. Two hundred people call the hot line.

THURSDAY, FEB. 9

Attendance at West High rebounds to about 80%.

The hot line gets 149 calls.

FRIDAY, FEB. 10

Three-year-old boy is discharged.

The hot line is deactivated.

MONDAY, FEB. 13

Osterholm announces that 100 Mankato West students are the key to the outbreak.

SUNDAY, FEB. 26

3 p.m. Ryan Pitt, 7, is admitted to the hospital with tentative diagnosis of meningitis.

MONDAY, FEB. 27

7:30 a.m. Community meeting is held to develop possible action plan to vaccinate preschool through sixth-grade children.

Hot line is reactivated; 103 calls received.

TUESDAY, FEB. 28

6:30 p.m. Community meeting held at Mankato West to discuss findings and plan.

Hot line gets 231 calls.

WEDNESDAY, MARCH 1

Vaccination clinics for preschoolers through sixth grade are scheduled for Friday and Monday.

Hot line gets 215 calls.

THURSDAY, MARCH 2

Mankato State University student Christopher Wilson, 18, is reported to be hospitalized in Twin Cities with meningitis.

Health team decides to vaccinate and give antibiotics to everyone in Mankato 29 years and younger—some 22,000 more people in all.

Hot line gets 1,310 calls.

FRIDAY, MARCH 3

6,000 people are immunized at Army Reserve Center in Mankato.

Three thousand hot line calls are received.

SATURDAY, MARCH 4

Thousands more are immunized. Hot line gets 1,207 calls.

SUNDAY, MARCH 5

5,600 people are immunized. Hot line gets 775 calls.

MONDAY, MARCH 6

5,000 people are immunized. Hot line gets 997 calls.

WEDNESDAY, MARCH 8

Hot line gets 89 calls. Hot line is deactivated.

Source: Nurse practitioner Jane Schwickert, Immanuel-St. Joseph's Hospital, Mankato.

APPENDIX D

Institute for Clinical Systems Integration Guidelines*

The following Appendix includes Health Care Guideline Summaries from the Institute for Clinical Systems Integration for:

- Preventive Services for Children
- Immunization
- Preventive Counseling and Education
- Preventive Services for Adults

Preamble

The central purpose of this guideline is to clearly identify those preventive services which are essential to provide to all low risk/asymptomatic members/patients on the basis of either *good* or *fair* evidence for inclusion in a periodic health evaluation (per USPSTF rules). A secondary purpose is to identify those services which should *not* be included in light of similarly strong evidence.

We recognize that many aspects of traditional periodic examinations, especially much of the traditional history and physical examination, will not be mentioned because they do not fall into either of the above categories. In some cases, this is because there is no evidence; in others, the evidence is conflicting or primarily anecdotal. We also recognize that changing these elements will be difficult for some providers and some patients. Therefore, we leave unaddressed components to the desires of individual medical groups while encouraging them to focus primarily on seeing that everyone gets the described essential components and eliminating services clearly of no overall value.

This guideline encompasses both preventive services and disease screening. The Preventive Guidelines Subcommittee used a multidisciplinary process and evidence-based methods to develop this guideline. This approach emphasizes the critical evaluation of scientific evidence, rather than expert opinion or consensus, to define necessary and appropriate care. Judging health benefit on the basis of scientific evidence provides a rational, defensible basis for directing resources toward effective preventive care and away from ineffective services or interventions for which risks may exceed benefits. When the scientific data are lacking or the evidence is equivocal, then a preference-based approach is recommended, allowing patients and providers to collectively make complex value judgments about specific preventive interventions.

*For further information and complete Guidelines contact the Institute for Clinical Systems Integration Guidelines, 8009 34th Avenue South, Suite 1200, Bloomington, MN 55425, Telephone (612) 883-7999, Fax (612) 858-9675, e-mail <icsi.info@healthpartners.com>

The proper selection of screening tests requires careful consideration of the age, sex, and other individual risk factors of the patient. Recommended screening tests must meet the following criteria:

a. Early diagnosis must be scientifically proven to lead to improved clinical outcome.
b. Additional resources must be available to confirm the diagnosis and provide care for those who screen positive.
c. Patients who are screened must be willing to comply with subsequent treatment recommendations.
d. The burden of disability from the target disease must warrant action.
e. The effectiveness of the individual components of the screening test must have been documented prior to their combination.
f. The cost, accuracy, and acceptability of the screening test must be adequate for the population to be screened.

Health Care Guideline

The information contained in this *ICSI Health Care Guideline* is intended primarily for health professionals and the following expert audiences:

- Physicians, nurses, and other health care professional and provider organizations
- Health plans, health systems, health care organizations, hospitals and integrated health care delivery systems
- Medical specialty and professional societies
- Researchers
- Federal, state and local government health care policy makers and specialists
- Employee benefit managers

This *ICSI Health Care Guideline* should not be construed as medical advice or medical opinion related to any specific facts or circumstances. If you are not one of the expert audiences listed above you are urged to consult a health care professional regarding your own situation and any specific medical questions you may have. In addition, you should seek assistance from a health care professional in interpreting this *ICSI Health Care Guideline* and applying it in your individual case.

This *ICSI Health Care Guideline* is designed to assist clinicians by providing an analytical framework for the evaluation and treatment of patients, and is not intended either to replace a clinician's judgment or to establish a protocol for all patients with a particular condition. An *ICSI Health Care Guideline* rarely will establish the only approach to a problem.

Copies of this *ICSI Health Care Guideline* may be distributed by any organization to the organization's employees but, except as provided below, may not be distributed outside of the organization without the prior written consent of the Institute for Clinical Systems Integration, Inc. If the organization is a legally constituted medical group, the *ICSI Health Care Guideline* may be used by the medical group in any of the following ways:

- Copies may be provided to anyone involved in the medical group's process for developing and implementing clinical guidelines
- The *ICSI Health Care Guideline* may be adopted or adapted for use within the medical group only, provided that ICSI receives appropriate attribution on all written or electronic documents
- Copies may be provided to patients and the clinicians who manage their care, if the *ICSI Health Care Guideline* is incorporated into the medical group's clinical guideline program

All other copyright rights in this *ICSI Health Care Guideline* are reserved by the Institute for Clinical Systems Integration, Inc. The Institute for Clinical Systems Integration, Inc. assumes no liability for any adaptations or revisions or modifications made to this *ICSI Health Care Guideline*.

Priority Aims for Medical Groups When Using This Guideline

1. Increase the percentage of patients who are up-to-date on preventive services.
Possible measures of accomplishing this aim:
a. Percentage of patients who are up-to-date on preventive services.

2. Increase the percentage of preventive services that are up-to-date.
Possible measures of accomplishing this aim:
a. Percentage of preventive services that are up-to-date.

3. Decrease the use of inappropriate screening maneuvers.
Possible measures of accomplishing this aim:
a. Percentage of children age 2 or under receiving lipids screening.
b. Percentage of patients (any selected group over the age of 2) receiving a routine urinalysis.
c. Percentage of patients (any selected group) having routine hemoglobin testing.

4. Increase the regular use of comprehensive health risk assessments.
Possible measures of accomplishing this aim:
a. Percentage of patients who have a current risk assessment tool in their medical record.
b. Percentage of patients who have a completed risk assessment tool in their medical record.

Preventive Services for Ages Birth–24 Months

Schedule of Visits:
First 2 weeks, 2, 4, 6–9, 15 months*
*Immunizations need to be given at 6 months.

Screening Maneuvers

- Risk assessment
- Interval history
- Developmental/ Behavioral assessment
- Appropriate physical examination at first encounter; per provider preference at subsequent encounters
- Head circumference
- Plotted height and weight
- Vision and hearing (by subjective assessment)
- Hemoglobin or hematocrit (once during infancy)

High-Risk Groups

- Tuberculin skin test (PPD)
- Blood lead testing (6 months to 6 years old)

- Neonatal screening (per state requirements)

Counseling & Education

Topics: Good Evidence

- Breast feeding
- Viral upper respiratory infection

Topics: Fair Evidence

- Iron rich diet
- Child safety seats
- Poison prevention
- Water heaters
- Flame-resistant sleepwear
- Infant sleep position and SIDS
- Infants & bottles

Topics: Insufficient Evidence

- Formula use
- Tobacco (incl. passive exposure)
- Motor vehicles/bicycles
- Fire safety
- Poison, water safety, and choking
- Falls, water heater safety
- Firearm storage
- Promotion of nonviolent behavior
- Coping skills/stress reduction
- Protection from UV light
- Preventive care visits
- Infants and bottles
- Fluoride supplements
- Wiping teeth with gauze
- Breast feeding

Immunizations and Chemoprophylaxis

- Diphtheria-tetanus-pertussis (DTP) vaccine: 2, 4, 6, 15 mos.
- Poliovirus vaccine (OPV or e-IPV): 2, 4, 6–15 mos.
- Measles-mumps-rubella vaccine (MMR): 12–15 mos.
- *Haemophilus influenzae* type b (Hib) conjugate vaccine: 2, 4, 6 (optional), 12–15 mos.
- Hepatitis B vaccine: birth–2 wks, 1–2 mos., 6–18 mos., OR 1–2 mos., 4 mos., 6–18 mos.
- Varicella vaccine: 12–18 mos.
- Rotavirus: 2, 4, 6 mos.

High-Risk Groups

- Influenza vaccine

Practices to Consider Discontinuing:

- Routine urinalysis
- Lipid screening under age 2
- Routine tuberculin skin test
- Routine blood chemistries

Preventive Services for Ages 2–6 Years

Schedule of Visits:
2 Years, 3–4 Years, 5 Years*
*The scheduling of the 2 year visit is left to the discretion of the clinician and the parent or guardian.

Screening Maneuvers	Counseling & Education	Immunizations & Chemoprophylaxis
■ Risk assessment ■ Interval history ■ Developmental/ Behavioral assessment ■ Physical examination per provider preference ■ Plotted height and weight ■ Vision and hearing (subjective) ■ Blood pressure ■ Eye examination for amblyopia and strabismus *High-Risk Groups* ■ Hearing ■ Tuberculin skin test (PPD) ■ Blood lead testing (6 months to 6 years old) ■ Lipid testing	**Topics: Fair Evidence** ■ Iron rich diet ■ Poison prevention ■ Water heaters ■ Flame-resistant sleepwear ■ Safety belts ■ Physical activity **Topics: Insufficient Evidence** ■ 5 a day (fruits and vegetables) ■ Parent role models ■ Healthy snacks ■ Calcium intake ■ Tobacco (incl. passive exposure) ■ Motor vehicles/bicycles ■ Fire safety ■ Poison, water safety, and choking ■ Falls, water heater safety ■ Firearm storage ■ Promotion of nonviolent behavior ■ Coping skills/stress reduction ■ Protection from UV light ■ Preventive care visits ■ Dental & periodontal disease	■ Diphtheria-tetanus-pertussis (DTP) vaccine (4–6 years old) ■ Oral poliovirus vaccine (OPV) (4–6 years old) ■ MMR booster (4–6 years old) *High-Risk Groups* ■ Hepatitis B vaccine ■ Influenza vaccine ■ Pneumococcal vaccine **Practices to Consider Discontinuing:** ■ Routine urinalysis ■ Routine hemoglobin testing ■ Routine tuberculin skin test ■ Routine blood chemistries

Preventive Services for Ages 7–12 Years

Schedule of Visits:
Ages 7–9, 12

Screening Maneuvers

- Risk assessments
- Interval history
- Developmental/Behavioral assessment
- Physical examination per provider preference
- Blood pressure
- Plotted height and weight

High-Risk Groups
- Tuberculin skin test (PPD)
- Lipid testing

Counseling & Education

Topics: Fair Evidence
- Poison prevention
- Water heaters
- Flame-resistant sleepwear
- Safety belts
- Safety helmets
- Physical activity

Topics: Insufficient Evidence
- 5 a day (fruits and vegetables)
- Food labels
- Parent role models
- Healthy snacks
- Calcium intake
- Alcohol and other drugs
- Tobacco (incl. passive exposure)
- Start of tobacco use
- Motor vehicles/bicycles
- Fire safety
- Poison, water safety, and choking
- Firearm storage
- Promotion of nonviolent behavior
- Coping skills/stress reduction
- Protection from UV light
- Preventive care visits
- Dental & periodontal disease

Immunizations & Chemoprophylaxis

- MMR booster (ages 5–12)
- Adult Td (age 12) if not previously done
- Hepatitis B

High-Risk Groups
- Influenza vaccine
- Pneumococcal vaccine

Practices to Consider Discontinuing:
- Routine urinalysis
- Routine hemoglobin testing
- Routine tuberculin skin test
- Routine blood chemistries

Preventive Services for Ages 13–18 Years

Schedule of Visits:
Two visits between ages 13 and 18*
*The scheduling of the second visit is left to the discretion of both the clinician and the parent or guardian.

Screening Maneuvers

- Risk assessment
- Interval history
- Developmental/ Behavioral assessment
- Physical examination per provider preference
- Plotted height and weight
- Blood pressure
- Papanicolaou smear (pelvic examination) (starting at age 18 or with onset of sexual activity—maximum interval, 3 yrs.)

High-Risk Groups

- Tuberculin skin test (PPD)
- Clinical testicular examination
- Sexually transmitted disease testing
- Lipid screening

Counseling & Education

Topics: Good Evidence

- Folic acid
- Limit dietary fat
- Tobacco cessation

Topics: Fair Evidence

- Caloric balance/nutrient balance
- Drinking and driving (good, fair)
- Safety belts (good, fair)
- Safety helmets
- Unintended pregnancy prevention
- Physical activity

Topics: Insufficient Evidence

- 5 a day (fruits and vegetables)
- Calcium intake
- Food labels
- Healthy snacks
- Tobacco (incl. passive exposure)
- Start of tobacco use
- Alcohol and other drugs
- Motor vehicle operation
- Motor vehicles/bicycles
- Helmets for motorcyclists (good, insufficient)
- Fire safety
- Firearm storage
- Promotion of nonviolent behavior
- STD prevention
- Depression/anxiety awareness
- Coping skills/stress reduction
- Protection from UV light
- Preventive care visits
- Preconception counseling
- Dental & periodontal disease

Immunizations & Chemoprophylaxis

- Hepatitis B vaccine

High-Risk Groups

- Influenza vaccine
- Pneumococcal vaccine

Practices to Consider Discontinuing:

- Routine urinalysis
- Routine hemoglobin testing
- Routine tuberculin skin test
- Routine blood chemistries

Immunizations

Routine Immunization Schedule for Infants and Children

Vaccine	2 mo	4 mo	6 mo	12 mo	15 mo	4–6 yr	12 yr
DTaP(1)	x	x	x		x	x	adult Td
Polio(2)	x	x	x			x	
MMR(3)					x	x	
Rotavirus(4)	x	x	x				
Varicella(5)					x		
Hib(6)	x	x	x (optional)	x			
Hepatitis B(7)	(see below)						

DTaP: Diphtheria and tetanus toxoids with acellular pertussis are preferred for all doses in the immunization schedule.

Polio: Live oral poliovirus vaccine (OPV), or enhanced-potency inactivated poliovirus vaccine (e-IPV). There are 3 acceptable schedule options, listed here in order of work group preference:

1. A sequential schedule of 2 eIPV at 2 and 4 months followed by 2 OPV at 6–15 months and 4–6 years;
2. 4 OPV at 2, 4, 6–15 months, and 4–6 years; or
3. 4 eIPV at 2, 4, and 6–15 months and 4–6 years.

MMR: Measles, mumps, rubella viruses in a combined vaccine. The second dose should be given from 4–6 years of age.

Rotavirus: Children born June through November may receive an accelerated schedule starting at 6 weeks of age and given every 3 weeks and completed by 3 months of age.

Varicella: Universal immunization of all infants without history of varicella is recommended at 12 to 18 months. Immunization should not be deferred past the age of 5 years.

Hib: 3 Hib conjugates are licensed for infant use. If PRP-OMP (Ped VaxHib from Merck) is given at 2 & 4 months, a dose at 6 months is not required.

For Vaccinations for High Risk Children (Pneumococcus, Influenza, Hepatitis A, Meningococcus) see annotations.(8)

Hepatitis B Immunization for Adults and Children(7)

HBV	1st Injection	2nd Injection	3rd Injection
Infants			
Schedule 1	at birth–2 weeks	1-2 mo old	6-18 mo old
Schedule 2	1-2 mo old	4 mo old	6-18 mo old
Adolescents & Adults			
Schedule 3	12–39 yrs old	1 mo after 1st	≥ 4 mo after 1st and ≥ 2 mo after 2nd

The standard for Hepatitis B immunization is universal vaccination of infants and vaccination of all adolescents and adults under 40 and adults of high risk who didn't receive immunization in infancy.

Adult Immunization Schedule - Routine and High Risk

Vaccine	19–39 Years	40–64 Years	65 Years & Older
Varicella(5)	Persons with no history of varicella, do titre. If negative, vaccinate.	-	-
Td(1)	Booster every 10 years	Booster every 10 years	Booster every 10 years
Influenza(9)	Annually between Oct–Dec for high risk groups	Annually between Oct–Dec for high risk groups	Annually
Pneumococcal(10)	Vaccinate high risk groups once. Revaccinate those at risk of losing immunity after 5 years.	Vaccinate high risk groups once. Revaccinate those at risk of losing immunity after 5 years.	Vaccinate at 65 if not done previously. Revaccinate if 1st received >5 years ago and before age 65.
Hepatitis A(11)	Risk groups.	Risk groups.	Risk groups.
Hepatitis B(7)	Universal vaccination if not done previously (see schedule above)	Risk groups.	Risk groups.
Lyme Disease(12)	Risk groups.	Risk groups.	Risk groups.
MMR(3)	Persons born after 1956 should have 2 doses measles; additional doses should be given as MMR.		

TB Testing(13)

Routine tuberculin skin testing of all patients is not necessary. High-risk groups identified in the algorithm annotations should be tested.

Testing is to be done as follows: 5 Tuberculin Units (TU) of Purified Protein Derivative (PPD) injected intradermally by standard "Mantoux" techniques.

Preventive Counseling and Education—by Topic

Birth to 24 Months	2 to 6 years	7 to 12 Years	13 to 18 Years	19 to 39 Years	40 to 64 Years	65+ Years	Topics/Subtopic
							1. Nutrition
•							Breastfeeding
•							Formula Use
•	•						Iron Rich Diet
	•	•					Parent Role Models
	•	•	•				Healthy Snacks
	•	•	•	•	•	•	Calcium Intake
•	•	•	•	•	•	•	Food Labels
			•	•			Folic Acid Supplements
			•	•	•		Limit Dietary Fat
	•	•	•	•	•	•	5 A Day (fruits and vegetables rich diet)
			•	•	•	•	Caloric Balance/Nutrient Balance
	•	•	•	•	•	•	**2. Physical Activity**
•	•	•	•	•	•	•	**3. Substance Use/Abuse**
•	•	•	•	•	•	•	Tobacco (includes passive exposure)
		•	•				Start of Tobacco Use
		•	•	•	•	•	Alcohol and Other Drugs
			•	•	•	•	Drinking and Driving Motor Vehicles
			•	•	•	•	Motor Vehicle Operations
							4. Injury Prevention
•							Child Safety Seats
•	•					•	Falls
•	•	•	•	•	•	•	Firearm Storage
•	•	•	•	•	•	•	Fire Safety
•	•	•					Flame Resistant Sleep Wear
			•	•	•	•	Helmet for Motorcycles
•	•	•	•	•	•	•	Motor Vehicles/Bicycles
•	•	•					Poison, Water Safety, Choking
	•	•	•	•	•	•	Safety Belts
		•	•				Safety Helmets
•	•					•	Water Heater Safety
							5. Violence and Abuse
•	•	•	•	•	•	•	Promotion of Non-Violent Behavior
							6. Sexual Practices
			•	•			Unintended Pregnancy Prevention
			•	•	•	•	STD Prevention

Birth to 24 Months	2 to 6 years	7 to 12 Years	13 to 18 Years	19 to 39 Years	40 to 64 Years	65+ Years	Topic/Subtopic (continued)
							7. Mental Health
			•	•	•	•	Depression/Anxiety Awareness
•	•	•	•	•	•	•	Coping Skills/Stress Reduction
				•	•	•	**8. Advance Directives**
					•		**9. Post Menopausal Hormone Prophylaxis**
							10. Skin Cancer
•	•	•	•	•	•	•	Protection from UV Light
•							**11. VURI Visits**
•							**12. Infant Sleep Positioning and SIDS**
•	•	•	•	•	•	•	**13. Preventive Care Visits**
			•	•	•		**14. Preconception Counseling**
•	•	•	•	•	•	•	**15. Dental and Periodontal Disease**
•							Infants and Bottles
•							Fluoride Supplements

Topics, Based on Strength of Recommendation

There is *good* evidence to support the recommendation that the condition be specifically considered in a periodic health examination.

Birth to 24 Months	2 to 6 years	7 to 12 Years	13 to 18 Years	19 to 39 Years	40 to 64 Years	65+ Years	Topic/Subtopic (continued)
							1. Nutrition
			•	•	•	•	Limit Dietary Fat
•							Breast Feeding
			•	•			Folic Acid Supplements
							3. Substance Use/Abuse
			•	•	•	•	Tobacco Cessation
				•	•	•	**8. Advance Directives**
•							**15. Viral Upper Respiratory Infection Visits**

There is *fair* evidence to support the recommendation that this condition be specifically considered in a periodic health examination.

Birth to 24 Months	2 to 6 years	7 to 12 Years	13 to 18 Years	19 to 39 Years	40 to 64 Years	65+ Years	Topic/Subtopic (continued)
							1. Nutrition
			•	•	•	•	Caloric Balance/Nutrient Balance
•	•						Iron Rich Diet
	•	•	•	•	•	•	**2. Physical Activity**
							3. Substance Use/Abuse
			•	•	•	•	Drinking and Driving Motor Vehicles
							4. Injury Prevention
•							Child Safety Seats
•	•	•					Poisoning Prevention
•	•	•					Water Heaters
•	•	•					Flame-Resistant Sleep Wear
	•	•	•	•	•	•	Safety Belts
		•	•				Safety Helmets
							6. Sexual Practices
			•	•			Unintended Pregnancy Prevention
					•		**9. Post Menopausal Hormone Prophylaxis**
•							**12. Infant Sleep Positioning and SIDS**
							14. Dental and Periodontal Disease
•							Infants and Bottles

This guideline pertains to the following age groups:

- 19 to 39 Years
- 40 to 64 Years
- 65 Years and Older

The following ICSI Preventive Sub-guidelines are referenced within the Preventive Services for Adults Guideline:

- Preventive Counseling and Education
- Tobacco Use Prevention and Cessation for Adults and Mature Adolescents
- Cervical Cancer Screening
- Adult Lipid Screening
- Colorectal Cancer Screening
- Immunizations
- Hormone Replacement Therapy

There is *insufficient* evidence to support the recommendation for or against the inclusion of the condition in a periodic health examination; however, the ICSI Preventive Counseling work group, based on their extensive clinical experience, recommend that counseling for these topics be included in a periodic health examination.

Birth to 24 Months	**2 to 6 years**	**7 to 12 Years**	**13 to 18 Years**	**19 to 39 Years**	**40 to 64 Years**	**65+ Years**	**Topic/Subtopic**
	•	•	•	•	•	•	**1. Nutrition**
		•	•	•	•	•	**5 A Day** (fruits and vegetables rich diet)
•							Food Labels
	•	•					Formula Use
	•	•	•				Parent Role Models
	•	•	•	•	•	•	Healthy Snacks
							Calcium Intake
							3. Substance Use/Abuse
•	•	•	•	•	•	•	Tobacco (incl. passive exposure)
		•	•				Start of Tobacco Use
		•	•	•	•	•	Alcohol and Other Drugs
			•	•	•	•	Motor Vehicle Operation
							4. Injury Prevention
•	•	•	•	•	•	•	Motor Vehicles/Bicycles
			•	•	•	•	Helmets for Motorcyclists
•	•	•	•	•	•	•	Fire Safety
•	•	•					Poison, Water Safety, Choking
•	•					•	Falls, Water Heater Safety
•	•	•	•	•	•	•	Firearm Storage
							5. Violence and Abuse
•	•	•	•	•	•	•	Promotion of Nonviolent Behavior
							6. Sexual Practices
			•	•	•	•	STD Prevention
							7. Mental Health
			•	•	•	•	Depression/Anxiety Awareness
•	•	•	•	•	•	•	Coping Skills/Stress Reduction
							10. Skin Cancer
•	•	•	•	•	•	•	Protection from UV Light
•	•	•	•	•	•	•	**12. Preventive Care Visits**
			•	•	•		**13. Preconception Counseling**
•	•	•	•	•	•	•	**14. Dental and Periodontal Disease**
•							Infants and Bottles
•							Fluoride Supplements

Preventive Services for Ages 19–39

Schedule of Visits:
Males: *Every 5 Years*
Females: *Every 3–5 Years*

Screening Maneuvers	Counseling & Education	Immunizations & Chemoprophylaxis
■ Risk assessment ■ Height and weight ■ Blood pressure ■ Clinical breast examination (every 3 years starting at age 20) ■ Total cholesterol and HDL-cholesterol ■ Papanicolaou smear (pelvic examination) (maximum interval every 3 years after 3 consecutive annual normals) *High-Risk Groups* ■ Sexually transmitted disease testing	**Topics: Good Evidence** ■ Limit dietary fat ■ Folic acid supplement ■ Tobacco cessation ■ Advance directives **Topics: Fair Evidence** ■ Caloric/nutrient balance ■ Drinking and driving ■ Safety belts ■ Unintended pregnancy prevention ■ Physical activity **Topics: Insufficient Evidence** ■ 5 a day (fruits and vegetables) ■ Calcium intake ■ Tobacco (incl. passive exposure) ■ Alcohol and other drugs ■ Motor vehicle operation and substance abuse ■ Motor vehicles/bicycles ■ Helmets for motorcyclists ■ Fire safety ■ Firearm storage ■ Promotion of nonviolent behavior ■ STD prevention ■ Depression/anxiety awareness ■ Coping skills/stress reduction ■ Protection from UV light ■ Preventive care visits ■ Preconception counseling ■ Dental & periodontal disease	■ Tetanus-diptheria (Td) booster (every 10 years) ■ Varicella (if negative titer in patient without history of varicella) ■ Hepatitis B vaccine (if not done previously) *High-Risk Groups* ■ Lyme disease ■ Pneumococcal vaccine (every 5 years) ■ Influenza vaccine (annually) ■ MMR 2nd dose ■ Hepatitis A vaccine **Practices to Consider Discontinuing:** ■ Routine hemoglobin testing ■ Routine blood chemistries ■ Routine urinalysis ■ Routine objective vision and hearing testing ■ Resting EKG ■ CA 125 & pelvic ultrasound for ovarian cancer screening

Preventive Services for Ages 40–64

Schedule of Visits:
Males: *Every 5 Years*
Females: *Every 3–5 Years*

Screening Maneuvers

- Risk assessment
- Height and weight
- Blood pressure
- Clinical breast examination (yearly)
- Total cholesterol and HDL-cholesterol
- Papanicolaou smear (pelvic examination) (maximum interval every 3 years after 3 consecutive annual normals)
- Mammogram (optional 40–49, yearly 50–75)
- Colon cancer screening

High-Risk Groups

- Sexually transmitted disease testing
- Diabetes screening

Counseling & Education

Topics: Good Evidence

- Limit dietary fat
- Tobacco cessation
- Advance directives

Topics: Fair Evidence

- Caloric/nutrient balance
- Drinking and driving (good and fair evidence)
- Safety belts
- Post menopausal hormone
- Prophylaxis
- Physical activity

Topics: Insufficient Evidence

- Food Labels
- 5 a day
- Calcium intake
- Tobacco (incl. passive exposure)
- Alcohol and other drugs
- Motor vehicle operation and substance abuse
- Motor vehicles/bicycles
- Helmets for motorcyclists
- Fire safety
- Firearm storage
- Promotion of nonviolent behavior
- STD prevention
- Depression/anxiety awareness
- Coping skills/stress reduction
- Protection from UV light
- Preventive care visits
- Preconception counseling
- Dental & periodontal disease

Immunizations & Chemoprophylaxis

- Tetanus-diptheria (Td) booster (every 10 years)

High-Risk Groups

- Hepatitis A vaccine
- Hepatitis B vaccine
- Pneumococcal vaccine (every 5 years)
- Influenza vaccine (annually)
- MMR
- Aspirin prophylaxis
- Lyme disease

Practices to Consider Discontinuing:

- Routine hemoglobin testing
- Routine blood chemistries
- Routine urinalysis
- Routine objective vision and hearing testing
- Resting EKG
- CA 125 & pelvic ultrasound for ovarian cancer screening
- DRE/Prostrate Specific Antigen for prostrate cancer screening

Preventive Services for Ages 65 and Over

Schedule of Visits:
Every 1–2 years

Screening Maneuvers

- Risk assessment
- Review medications
- Height and weight
- Blood pressure
- Clinical breast examination
- Total cholesterol and HDL-cholesterol
- Colon cancer screening
- Papanicolaou smear (pelvic examination may be performed at the mutual consent of the patient and provider after age 65)
- Mammogram (annually until age 75)
- Objective visual acuity testing (after age 74)
- Subjective hearing testing (after age 74)

High-Risk Groups
- Diabetes screening

Counseling & Education

Topics: Good Evidence
- Limit dietary fat
- Tobacco cessation
- Advance directives

Topics: Fair Evidence
- Caloric/nutrition balance
- Drinking and driving (good and fair evidence)
- Safety belts (good, fair)
- Post menopausal hormone
- Prophylaxis
- Physical activity

Topics: Insufficient Evidence
- 5 a day (fruits and vegetables)
- Food labels
- Calcium intake
- Tobacco (incl. passive exposure)
- Alcohol and other drugs
- Motor vehicle operation and substance abuse
- Motor vehicles/bicycles
- Helmets for motorcyclists
- Fire safety
- Falls, water heater safety
- Firearm storage
- Promotion of nonviolent behavior
- STD prevention
- Depression/anxiety awareness
- Coping skills/stress reduction
- Protection from UV light
- Preventive Care visits
- Dental & periodontal disease

Immunizations & Chemoprophylaxis

- Tetanus-diptheria (Td) booster (every 10 years)
- Influenza vaccine (annually)
- Pneumococcal vaccine (every 5 years)

High-Risk Groups
- Hepatitis A vaccine
- Hepatitis B vaccine
- Aspirin prophylaxis
- Lyme disease

Practices to Consider Discontinuing:
- Routine hemoglobin testing
- Routine blood chemistries
- Routine urinalysis
- Routine objective vision and hearing testing up to age 75
- Resting EKG
- CA 125 & pelvic ultrasound for ovarian cancer screening
- DRE/Prostate Specific Antigen for prostate cancer screening

INDEX